D0262297

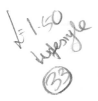

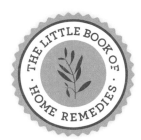

THE LITTLE BOOK OF · HOME REMEDIES ·

MIND
— and —
BODY

Natural Recipes for
Peace of Mind

Linda B. White, M.D.
Barbara H. Seeber & Barbara Brownell Grogan

First published in the USA in 2015 by
Fair Winds Press, a member of
Quarto Publishing Group USA Inc.
100 Cummings Center
Suite 406-L
Beverly, MA 01915-6101
www.fairwindspress.com
Visit www.bodymindbeautyhealth.com. It's your personal guide to a happy, healthy,
and extraordinary life!

19 18 17 16 15   1 2 3 4 5

ISBN: 978-1-59233-672-2

Content for this book was previously published in the book *500 Time-Tested Home
Remedies and the Science Behind Them* by Linda B. White, M.D., Barbara Brownell
Grogan, and Barbara H. Seeber (Fair Winds Press, 2014).

Cover design by Leigh Ring // RingArtDesign.com
Book design by Leigh Ring // RingArtDesign.com

The information in this book is for educational purposes only. It is not intended to
replace the advice of a physician or medical practitioner. Please see your health care
provider before beginning any new health program. The authors and publisher are
not responsible for readers' misuse of these recipes and, as a result, any unintended
effects.

Printed and bound in the USA

Contents

Introduction... 4

Brain Health.. 6

Depression... 16

Fatigue.. 24

High Blood Pressure....................................... 34

Immune System Support.................................... 42

Indigestion and Irritable Bowel System Support . 50

Insomnia... 60

Menopause... 68

Morning Sickness.. 76

Premenstrual Syndrome.................................... 84

Prostate Health.. 92

Stress and Anxiety.. 102

Ulcers... 110

Vaginal Yeast Infections.................................. 118

Introduction

In today's high-powered, health-conscious world, we're all smarter, more informed about our bodies, and preoccupied with ways to live long, healthy lives. We've accomplished half of that goal: living longer. But we're missing the "living healthier" part of the equation.

On December 15, 2012, the British medical journal *The Lancet* published data from the Global Burden of Disease Study 2010. Here are the key findings, starting with the good news: Around the world, longevity has increased. We're less likely to succumb prematurely to malaria and measles, but more likely to drop dead later in life from heart attack or stroke. The bad news is, we're more likely to spend our last years disabled by diseases—most of which are preventable.

Chronic illness has long dogged Americans. Now it's spreading to other countries. Where have we gone wrong? We have health-related facts and figures at our fingertips. We have expensive diagnostic tests, highly trained doctors, and cutting-edge treatments. The shelves in supermarkets groan under the weight of boxes, cans, and bags. Modern conveniences have reduced our need for physical labor. Computers give us up to-date medical bulletins.

Despite these advances, and to some extent because of them, we've become fat, flabby, and frequently ill. We're too often hurried, harried, sleep-deprived, and socially disconnected. We eat in our cars, at our desks, in front of televisions—everywhere but at the dining room table in the company of others. We sit too much and move too little.

It turns out that health springs largely from old-fashioned behaviors—eating wholesome food, enjoying friends, relaxing, getting enough sleep, moving our bodies, and using natural remedies to heal.

The goal of this book is to help you get back to the basic lifestyle measures that point you toward a healthy, vibrant future.

We provide lots of practical information on preventing and managing ailments. You'll find time-tested recipes and lifestyle tips all designed to give you sometimes quick, always natural, ways to soothe, calm, and heal.

We hope you enjoy this book. May it enlighten you, guiding you along natural and simple paths to your healthy future.

Brain Health

A 2013 study showed that women who've crossed the menopause threshold experience subtle declines in cognitive function. These skills include learning, remembering, problem-solving, and paying attention. Before you beg your doctor for a prescription for hormones, know that (1) the early menopause brain fog is transient; (2) the long-term effects of menopause on mental function are negligible; and (3) hormone replacement doesn't seem to help and may, in fact, worsen cognitive performance.

For men and women, rates of dementia rise with age. According to the Centers for Disease Control and Prevention, the risk of Alzheimer's disease (the most common type of dementia) doubles every five years for people over age sixty-five. By age eighty-five, between 25 and 50 percent of people have signs of the disease.

Does that mean that if you live long enough, you're destined to develop dementia? Certainly not! Dementia is a disease, not a normal age change. It's marked by the progressive deterioration of memory, other intellectual functions, and the ability to perform daily tasks. The other most common type of dementia is vascular dementia (also called multi-infarct dementia), a condition that occurs when blood clots in brain arteries destroy small areas of tissue.

How do you know if memory loss is normal? Some degree of age-related forgetfulness happens to almost everyone. Whereas long-term memory (the names of your loved ones, significant events from your past) is normally well preserved, short-term memory gets a bit fuzzier. For instance, you may remember exactly what you were doing when you learned about the terrorist attacks on September 11, 2001, but forget where you put your car keys, why you walked into a room, or the name of the actor in the movie you saw last week. People with dementia forget big things: the names of close friends, how to balance a checkbook, or how to navigate from home to grocery store.

Research has shown that some two-thirds of memory-zapping aging can be attributed to lifestyle. This means there's a lot you can do to "head" it off!

Simple Salmon

If you remember to eat just this fish, you may find the adage, "Seafood is brain food" may turn out to be true.

1 pound (455 g) salmon fillet, or 4 fillets
(4 ounces, or 115 g each)

Freshly ground black pepper (optional)

1 tablespoon (15 ml) olive oil

1 teaspoon (1 g) crushed fresh oregano

1 lemon, cut into wedges

PREPARATION AND USE:

Preheat the oven to 450°F (230°C, or gas mark 8). Wash the fillet(s) and pat dry. Place the fish skin down on a baking sheet. Sprinkle with pepper, if using. In a small bowl, mix the olive oil and oregano. Brush this mixture onto the salmon. Bake for 10 to 15 minutes until flaky. Serve with the lemon wedges.

YIELD: 4 servings

❓ How it works: People who eat more cold-water fish, which is rich in the brain-friendly fatty acid docosahexaenoic acid (DHA), reduce their risk of cognitive decline and dementia. Fatty fish is also one of the few food sources of vitamin D, a vitamin with multiple functions, including proper brain function and nerve protection. Many Americans have insufficient blood levels of this vitamin. Unfortunately, low levels correlate with dementia.

Spicy Milk

I learned about this remedy while interviewing a National Institutes of Health pharmacologist for a story on herbs that protect against dementia.
~ LBW

1 teaspoon (2 g) ground turmeric

1/2 teaspoon freshly ground black pepper 1 cup (235 ml) whole milk

PREPARATION AND USE:

Mix the turmeric and pepper into the milk. Drink one serving twice daily—morning and evening.

YIELD: 1 Serving

? How it works: The key ingredient in curry is turmeric. It contains the potent anti-inflammatory and antioxidant agent curcumin, which may help to counter the inflammation and oxidation that promotes nerve-degenerating conditions such as dementia. Furthermore, cur-cumin inhibits the formation of beta-amyloid and improves its clearance. However, cur-cumin isn't well absorbed from the intestine. Consuming it with fat (as in full-fat milk, butter, or oil) and pepper improves absorption.

Berry Strong Brain

This sweet dessert salad will not disappoint your taste buds or brain cells.

1 cup (150 g) halved red grapes

1 cup (160 g) halved strawberries

1 cup (145 g) blackberries or blueberries

½ cup (87 g) pomegranate arils (sometimes called seeds)

½ cup (87 g) dark chocolate chips (optional)

Plain or honey-flavored Greek yogurt, for topping

PREPARATION AND USE:

Mix the grapes and berries in a large bowl. Stir in the pomegranate arils. Fold in the chocolate chips, if using. Divide among four dessert plates. Top each serving with a dab of yogurt.

YIELD: 4 servings

How it works: Berries, red grapes, pomegranate, and chocolate are rich in chemicals called polyphenols, which are antioxidant and anti-inflammatory. Regular consumption of berries is associated with a reduced risk of Parkinson's disease, which can cause dementia. In the cellular equivalent of housekeeping, extracts of strawberries and blueberries help the brain cells clean up toxic debris. In rats, a diet high in extracts of strawberries, blueberries, and blackberries reverses age-related deficits in learning and memory. Grape polyphenols reduce production of beta amyloid, inhibit its tendency to clump, protect the brain cells from its toxic effects, and curb inflammatory activity.

Note: To peel and remove the arils from a pomegranate, see http://mideastfood.about.com/od/tipsandtechniques/ss/deseedpomegrana_2.htm. Also, for a superfast, nonwater removal, go to http://vimeo.com/39205407.

Moroccan Sage Tea

This traditional drink is popular in Morocco in the winter months. It gives brain-healthy benefits throughout the year.

1 teaspoon (2 g) green tea leaves

1 teaspoon (1 g) dried sage

2 cups (475 ml) boiling water

Stevia, to taste

PREPARATION AND USE:

Place the tea leaves and sage in a teapot. Pour the boiling water over the mixture. Steep for 5 minutes. Gently stir the tea and strain into two cups. Add stevia.

YIELD: 2 servings

? How it works: Lab experiments show green tea polyphenols are antioxidant and nerve protectant and inhibit beta-amyloid–induced nerve damage. Populations that drink more green tea have been found to have a lower rate of cognitive impairment. Chemicals in garden sage are anti-inflammatory and antioxidant, help preserve the brain's acetylcholine (a brain chemical decreased in Alzheimer's), and protect neurons from beta-amyloid's toxic effects. Several studies demonstrate memory enhancement with oral consumption of either dried leaf extracts or small amounts of diluted essential oil in healthy people, both old and young. At least one study shows that inhalation of the essential oil improves memory and mood.

Mind-Enhancing Hot Chocolate

Throw out that instant hot chocolate and rediscover the wonders in the cocoa powder your mom used.

1 cup (235 ml) almond milk

2 tablespoons (10 g) unsweetened cocoa powder

½ teaspoon vanilla extract

Pinch of salt

Stevia (we use ½ packet [0.5 g]), equivalent to 1 teaspoon [4 g] sugar)

Pinch of ground cinnamon

PREPARATION AND USE:

In a medium-size saucepan, mix together the almond milk, cocoa powder, vanilla extract, and salt. Warm over low heat. Add stevia to taste. Whisk as the mixture warms until it is frothy and steaming. Pour into a cup and top with the cinnamon. If it's too thick for your taste, try adding up to ½ cup (120 ml) of water.

YIELD: 1 serving

❓ How it works: Consumption of another polyphenol-rich food, chocolate, has been shown to reduce the risk of stroke. A dose of cocoa increased blood flow to the brain's gray matter while healthy volunteers took a cognitive test. In one study, 90 seniors with mild cognitive impairment drank cocoa with varying amounts of flavanols (a polyphenol) for eight weeks. Those with the higher amounts in their drink tested with improved attention and other mental skills.

Mental Focus Aromatherapy
(or, Think Sharp Scents)

This delightfully scented remedy enhances memory.

1 drop sage essential oil

2 drops rosemary essential oil

3 drops peppermint essential oil

PREPARATION AND USE:

In a small, clean jar, blend the sage, rosemary, and peppermint oils. Drop a cotton ball into the jar. Apply the essential oils to the cotton ball. Cap tightly. Open the jar and sniff daily.

YIELD: A week's worth of sniff sessions

❓ **How it works:** Studies show that among essential oils, sage, rosemary, and peppermint all enhance memory.

LIFESTYLE TIP

Crack open a Brazil nut. Brazil nuts are rich in selenium, a mineral that acts as an antioxidant and contributes to normal brain functions. Scientists have linked higher selenium levels in the body with a lower risk of depression. Preliminary research suggests that low selenium is a risk factor for cognitive decline. Brown rice, oatmeal, and whole-grain breads are other good sources of selenium.

Riddle Me This

Mentally stimulating leisure activities, such as doing crossword puzzles, seem to help keep the brain sharp.

1 crossword or Sudoku puzzle

A pencil

PREPARATION AND USE:

Complete a puzzle per day.

YIELD: 1 challenge daily

❓ **How it works:** Studies show that activities that flex your mental power may delay mental decline with age, possibly by building the brain's reserve capacity. In a 2011 study, researchers compared seniors who regularly worked crossword puzzles ("puzzlers") to those who didn't (the "nonpuzzlers"). The puzzlers delayed the onset of accelerated memory loss (a sign of dementia) by an average of 2.54 years. In 2009, the same research group found that greater participation in a variety of mentally stimulating activities—puzzles, writing, playing board or card games, playing music, and participating in group discussions—delayed memory decline.

A Fast Walk to Clear Your Head

Do this every day to heighten awareness, take in vitamin D, and boost brain health.

1 pair walking shoes

You

PREPARATION AND USE:

Walk daily outside for 30 minutes. Identify a safe route and let yourself go; you'll find you are solving problems and thinking creatively as you become healthy and fit. For a vitamin D boost, walk 15 minutes without sunscreen and then slather it on your face, neck, and arms for the second half of your walk.

YIELD: 1 session daily

❓ **How it works:** Repeated studies show that regular exercise enhances learning and memory, improves vascular function, and helps prevent diseases such as diabetes and heart disease, both of which negatively affect the brain. Furthermore, physical activity lessens the impact of aging on the brain, as well as all other organ systems. It's never too late to start. A 2013 study published in the Journal of Aging Research demonstrated that, in seniors who already had mild cognitive impairment (a condition that's less severe than outright dementia), twice-weekly exercise—particularly aerobic exercise—improved memory. Walking halfway without sunscreen adds a vitamin D boost.

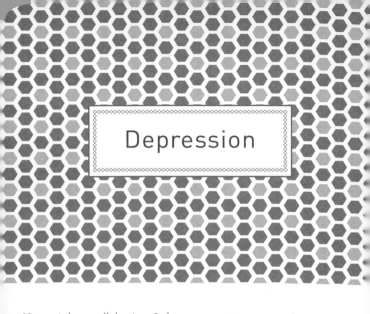

Depression

No one is happy all the time. Sadness represents an appropriate response to misfortune. For the psychologically hardy, low moods soon lift. Significant loss, however, produces grief, which can endure for months (for some people, depression can complicate normal grief). Barring tragedy, most people experience episodes of low mood against a backdrop of psychological well-being.

Depression isn't part of the normal emotional fabric. It burdens people with persistent unhappiness and an inability to derive pleasure from activities, even those that once brought joy. As opposed to "the blues," it impairs a person's ability to function.

This debilitating illness is all too common. According to the World Health Organization, depression affects 121 million people around the globe and places second behind heart disease as a leading cause of disability. About 16.3 million Americans over the age of eighteen experience some type of depression. Major depression strikes 20 percent of women and 13 percent of men.

This illness does more than engender sadness. Depressed people often feel irritable, angry, worthless, and ashamed. Thinking becomes irrationally negative. ("Nothing's any good. I'm a burden. I'll never get better.") Physical symptoms include increased pain, changes in appetite, and sleep disturbances.

In addition to major depression, other depressive illnesses include seasonal affective disorder (depression during the short days of winter), premenstrual dysphoria (depression around the time of menses), dysthymia (low-level depression that endures for at least two years), and bipolar disorder (formerly called manic depression and marked by alternating episodes of depression and mania).

Major depression is a serious illness. Not only does it diminish quality of life, but it raises the risk for chronic conditions such as heart disease and stroke. Like any other disease, it warrants professional treatment. The following recipes and tips are designed to buoy normal bouts of low mood and prevent depression. Please do not use these remedies as a substitute for professional treatment. If you think you are clinically depressed, get help.

Sunny Mediterranean Salad

1 cup (100 g) halved and pitted black olives

1 cup (100 g) halved and pitted green olives

1 cup (150 g) halved cherry tomatoes

1 cup (135 g) cubed cucumber

¼ cup (38 g) crumbled feta cheese

½ cup (60 g) crushed walnuts

½ teaspoon minced fresh garlic

Freshly ground black pepper

1 tablespoon (15 ml) extra-virgin olive oil

PREPARATION AND USE:

Mix together the olives, tomatoes, cucumber, and feta in a large bowl. Toss in the walnuts, garlic, and pepper to taste. Drizzle the olive oil over the salad and give it one final toss.

YIELD: 4 side salads

❓ **How it works:** One study found that women who ate a "traditional" diet (i.e., high in vegetables, fruit, meat, fish, and whole grains and low in sugar and processed foods) had lower odds of depression and anxiety. The inverse relationship was true for women who followed a "Western" diet (i.e., high in processed or fried foods, refined carbohydrates, sugary foods, and beer). People who follow a Mediterranean diet—a traditional diet that emphasizes vegetables, fruits, nuts, whole grains, fish, and olive oil—enjoy some protection against depression.

Good-Fat Fish

4 salmon, tuna, or herring fillets (3 ounces, or 85 g)

4 tablespoons (60 ml) olive oil, divided

Freshly ground black pepper

Juice of 1 lemon

2 tablespoons (22 g) Dijon mustard

Tabasco sauce

1 teaspoon (7 g) honey

¼ cup (16 g) chopped fresh dill

Lemon wedges, for garnish

PREPARATION AND USE:

Brush the salmon with 1 to 2 tablespoons (15 to 30 ml) of the olive oil
and season with the pepper. Broil for 3 to 4 minutes on each side, so that
the skin is brown and firm like meat. In a small bowl, whisk together the
remaining olive oil with the lemon juice, mustard, Tabasco sauce to taste,
honey, and dill. Add pepper to taste. Drizzle the sauce over the warm fillets
and serve with the lemon wedges.

YIELD: 4 servings

❓ **How it works:** Oily fish, such as tuna, salmon, herring, and mackerel,
are rich in the omega-3 fatty acids your brain needs to function properly. In
susceptible people, low levels seem to increase the risk of depression.

Cobra Pose

The cobra pose, called bhujangasana (boo-jang-ahhs-anna) in Sanskrit, is one of a series of heart-opening yoga exercises. Although such poses are practiced to help strengthen the back, tone the abdomen, and open the chest, they are also intended to balance the body and spirit.

You

Comfortable clothes

A pad or rug

PREPARATION AND USE:

Lie on your belly. Straighten your legs behind you. Draw your heels and toes together. Press your toenails and pubic bone against the ground. Rest your forehead on the floor. Place your palms against the floor, fingertips spread, hands facing forward. Hug your elbows to your sides (like cricket wings). Push down with your hands and arms so that your head, neck, and shoulders lift. All the while, keep your shoulders open, not hunched; keep your lower abdominals engaged to avoid pinching your lower back; and keep your neck in a neutral position. Breathe slowly in and out three to five times. Lower your body. Rest. Repeat three more times.

YIELD: 1 session

? How it works: Emerging research shows that yoga improves mood in people without bona fide depression. In people with major depression, the addition of yoga to antidepressant medications further reduces symptoms. Also, it's a big boost just being part of a class and enjoying the socialization it brings.

! Warning: Do not try this if you have a hernia, lower back pain, or are pregnant.

B-eautiful Crab Cakes

16 ounces (455 g) crabmeat, flaked

1 large egg, lightly beaten

1 cup (115 g) bread crumbs

¼ cup (25 g) scallion

¼ cup (60 g) plain low-fat Greek yogurt

1 teaspoon (5 ml) fresh lemon juice

1 tablespoon (15 ml) Worcestershire sauce

½ teaspoon minced fresh garlic

Freshly ground black pepper

Olive oil

PREPARATION AND USE:

In a large bowl, mix together all the ingredients until combined. Roll and shape the mixture into eight cakes. Coat a large skillet with a small amount of olive oil and place over medium-low heat. Cook the cakes until golden brown, about 3 minutes on each side.

YIELD: 4 servings

❓ How it works: It's easy to have a vitamin B12 deficiency if you don't consume animal foods: fish, meat, poultry, and eggs. Long-term vitamin B12 deficiency can lead to anemia, nerve damage, depression, memory loss, disorientation, and dementia. Crab is high in vitamin B12. Look for stone crabs and Dungeness, which are lowest in contaminants.

Aroma Lift

Your favorite uplifting plant essential oil

PREPARATION AND USE:

You can use essential oils in a variety of ways:

- Create blends or use them singly.
- Put a few drops in a commercial diffuser (which gently heats the oil to aerosolize the oils).
- If you don't have a diffuser, pour hot water into a bowl, add 3 drops of essential oil, and place nearby.
- You can also add 10 drops per ounce (28 ml) of unscented lotion or body oi
- Finally, you can add 10 drops to a bath and mix well.

YIELD: 1 application each

❓ **How it works:** Plant essential oils bind to receptors in the nose. Nerve impulses for smell affect areas related to mood. Also, aromas are linked to memories. The small molecules in plant essential oils can also cross the skin and the respiratory linings (when you inhale the airborne chemicals) to enter the bloodstream. In a study of depressed and anxious pregnant women, a diluted blend of rose and lavender improved symptoms. Centuries of use and preliminary studies indicate that other essential oils can positively modulate mood.

Note: Essential oil options include lemon, neroli, geranium, bergamot, clary sage, rose, lemon verbena, ylang ylang, jasmine, lavender, basil, and marjoram. (Avoid synthetic perfumes.) If you don't have any of these plant essential oils at home, go to the nearest natural food stores and sniff the sample bottles until you find a scent you enjoy. If the smell reminds you of a happy experience, that's exactly what you want.

Mindful Massage

2 tablespoons (30 ml) unscented lotion or vegetable oil

10 to 12 drops lavender essential oil, or your favorite

PREPARATION AND USE:

In a serene setting with your favorite calming music, slowly and deliberately add the lotion to a teacup. Drop in the essential oil. Mix with a spoon or chopstick. Dip one hand into the lotion and massage it into the opposite arm, thinking about the smooth feel of the lotion against your skin, the aroma of lavender, and the joy of the motion. When finished, pause. Appreciate your bodily sensations and the setting. Now massage your opposite arm, then each hand, leg, and foot, focusing on the slow, soothing motion of the massage and the velvety feel of the lotion against your skin. Take an appreciative pause as you finish each body part. Finish with your face, neck, and chest. Close your eyes for a few moments, inhaling and exhaling slowly.

YIELD: 1 application

❓ How it works: Mindfulness, by definition, helps you focus on the present moment, which can stop you from brooding. It can also help you appreciate the beauty around you. In a study involving pregnant women, mindfulness reduced symptoms of depression and facilitated maternal-infant bonding.

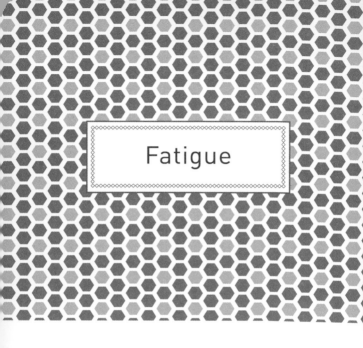

Fatigue

Far too many Americans drag through their days feeling weary and downright exhausted. In a survey of American workers, 38 percent reported feeling fatigued within a two-week period.

In a 2005 survey of 4,500 male and female twins, about 37 percent of the people reported extreme fatigue at some point in their lives. In addition, nearly 23 percent had experienced prolonged fatigue (longer than one month), and almost 16 percent had chronic fatigue (lasting more than six months). The women were two to three times more likely to feel run down as men. Specifically, 75 percent of the women reported fatigue, versus 25 percent of the men. The women also developed "fatiguing illness" at younger ages. We'll leave it up to our readers to speculate on why women are more vulnerable, though differences in genetics, hormones, and social demands (working and caring for family) could certainly be factors.

The most common reasons for feeling worn out are sleeping too little and being overscheduled—two familiar and coexisting problems in America. Another related issue is chronic stress overload, which leads to burnout (emotional detachment, apathy, and low energy). Ill-advised yet common solutions to coping with stress by eating junk food, smoking, or drinking heavily only compound the problem.

Fatigue can be physical, mental, and emotional. Repetitive activities in any one dimension can tire you out. If you exercised harder or longer than usual, you'll feel physically depleted. If you've been problem-solving for hours, your head will feel fuzzy. Staring endlessly at a computer screen fatigues the eyes. If you've been upset or have been comforting someone else, you may feel emotionally spent. The solution to overdoing it is to give yourself breaks.

Fatigue is a normal reaction to taxing your-self. If you feel better after you relax and get a good night's sleep, you're okay. Nevertheless, you should take care not to wear yourself out very often.

Sweet Pot-assium Energy Push

2 quarts (2 L) water

4 large sweet potatoes

2 tablespoons (30 g) plain Greek yogurt

1 teaspoon (5 ml) olive oil

Freshly ground black pepper

1 tablespoon (20 g) honey or agave nectar (optional)

PREPARATION AND USE:

Heat the water in a large pot over medium heat. Peel the potatoes and cut them into chunks. Add the chunks to the hot water and simmer until tender, about 20 minutes. Reduce the heat to low. Drain the potatoes, place back in the pan, and return the pan to the low heat. Mix the yogurt and olive oil until completely blended. Mash the potatoes, adding the yogurt mixture and mashing until smooth. Add pepper to taste. If desired, mix in honey to taste. Serve warm.

YIELD: 4 servings

❓ **How it works:** If your system is low in major nutrients, such as potassium, you'll feel the fatigue. Give your system an energy boost with potassium-rich veggies and fruits. Sweet potatoes, avocados, baked potatoes with their skin, edamame, and papayas deliver up to a whopping 1,000 milligrams per serving out of the recommended daily intake of 4,700 milligrams.

Breakfast Boost Omelet

Handful of well-rinsed baby spinach or kale

3 large or 4 small shiitake mushrooms

2 teaspoons (10 ml) olive oil

2 large eggs

1 tablespoon (15 ml) milk

Pinch of dried or fresh thyme and ground black pepper

PREPARATION AND USE:

Wash and pat dry the leafy greens. Tear into bite-size pieces, removing any thick stems. Wash, dry, and slice the mushrooms. Heat the oil in an omelet pan over medium heat. Sauté the mushrooms until they soften and brown. Scramble the eggs and milk in a bowl. Stir in the thyme and pepper. Pour over the mushrooms. When the center begins to gel, turn with a spatula to cook the other side, 2 to 3 minutes. Place the greens on one side of the omelet and fold the omelet in half. Remove from the pan and serve.

YIELD: 1 serving

How it works: You literally need to break your overnight fast in the morning. If you find yourself crashing before lunch, a nutritious breakfast might be the solution. The olive oil and the protein in the eggs supply long-lasting energy. (Cereal and baked goods, particularly if made from refined grains, give you a quick boost followed by a quick decline in blood glucose.) Leafy greens contain a host of vitamins, including calcium, magnesium, and B vitamins—all of which are needed in energy processes. Shiitakes contain fiber, minerals (potassium, magnesium, selenium), the B vitamin folate, and, when grown under ultraviolet light, vitamin D. They also taste delicious and promote immune health.

Pick-Me-Up Snack

If your energy sags between meals, try this healthy snack.

1 apple, cored and sliced

1 tablespoon (16 g) peanut butter

1 large carrot, sliced lengthwise

1 hard-boiled large egg

Freshly ground black pepper

PREPARATION AND USE:

Put dabs of peanut butter on the apple and carrot slices. Shell the egg and sprinkle with pepper. Enjoy and face your next few hours with energy.

YIELD: 1 serving

❓ **How it works:** Fatigue can result from eating too little and eating the wrong things. For instance, sweets cause a brisk but transient spike in blood sugar, but provide few nutrients. Instead, choose whole-food snacks, such as hard-boiled eggs, nuts, peanuts, carrots, and apples, which provide calories and the vitamins and minerals needed for energy production. Fresh fruits and vegetables are high in vitamin C and other antioxidants which counter the free radicals that lead to oxidative stress, which has been linked to fatigue. Antioxidants counter that effect. In a 2012 study, an intravenous infusion of vitamin C (not something to try at home) reduced fatigue in office workers.

Water on Hand

If you are thirsty, you're already dehydrated—a cause for fatigue. Drink up.

Fresh purified water

Lemon slices, crushed fresh mint, or cucumber slices

PREPARATION AND USE:

Pour water into a glass or, if you're on the go, a bottle. Add zing to the taste by adding one of the suggested options.

YIELD: 1 serving

❓ How it works: One symptom of dehydration is fatigue. Staying hydrated helps. And if you add lemon slices or lemon juice to your water, you're adding vitamin C and flavonoids that are also antioxidant. Drink at least eight 8-ounce (235 ml) glasses of water a day and more when you're active. Drink when you're thirsty. (The elderly may need help getting the amount they need because they don't have acute thirst sensation.) Go for two glasses in the morning, two glasses an hour before physical activity, sipping during the activity, and another two glasses afterward. Drink your other glasses in the late morning and early evening. Avoid drinking water 2 hours before bedtime, so you'll sleep the night through. You'll know you're getting enough water if you're urinating four to seven times a day. If you urinate less and your urine looks dark, you're probably dehydrated.

Iron Out Fatigue: Easy, Yummy Clams

Iron helps battle anemia, a major cause of fatigue. Women who menstruate heavily are at particular risk. A simple blood test can establish whether you need extra iron.

3 dozen clams (these can be little- or medium-neck)

3 tablespoons (42 g) unsalted butter

2 garlic cloves, minced

1 small onion, diced

½ cup (120 ml) white wine

¼ cup (15 g) chopped fresh parsley

Freshly ground black pepper

Lemon wedges, for garnish

Loaf of crusty whole wheat bread, sliced

PREPARATION AND USE:

Thoroughly wash the clams, throwing away any that have an odor. Over medium heat, melt the butter in a large pan. Add the garlic and onion and braise for about 3 minutes; do not allow them to burn. Pour in the wine and stir well. Increase the heat to medium-high and cook until the wine boils. Add the clams. Cover the pan and steam the clams, stirring occasionally, for 8 to 10 minutes, until they open. Throw away any clams that are still closed: they are likely bad. Toss in the fresh parsley, sprinkle the clams and broth with pepper, and stir the clams once more. Transfer the clams to a large serving bowl. Pour the clam broth over them and serve the clams steaming hot, garnished with lemon wedges. Serve with the bread: it's perfect for sopping up the clam broth.

YIELD: 4 appetizer servings

? How it works: Although beef liver and chicken liver top the list for iron-rich sources, shellfish is a major contender. Clams, oysters, and mussels have the same amount—about 3.5 milligrams per serving, (about eight clams). Spinach and dark leafy greens, beans, and tofu are among the best vegetable-based iron sources.

LIFESTYLE TIP

Stop smoking and stay away from others' smoke. In addition to many other toxic substances, tobacco smoke contains carbon monoxide, which reduces the oxygen-carrying capacity of your blood.

Mini Work Break

If you can't take a 10-minute break, short exercises can "reset" your brain.

You

Your office or cubicle

A chair

PREPARATION AND USE:

Energize One: Wall Tap: Stand up and touch one wall, and then walk to the other and touch it.

Energize Two: Arm Wrap: Stand up and wrap your left arm over your right, crossing your palms, too. Raise your elbows to shoulder height and press your palms away from your face. Hold for 10 to 20 seconds. Repeat on the other side.

Energize Three: Leg Wrap: Sitting at your desk, lift your feet and cross your right leg over the left. Repeat on the other side.

Energize Four: Infinity Trace: Extend your right arm in front of you. Hold out your thumb and trace the infinity sign (a sideways figure eight). Follow the motion with your eyes, without moving your head. Repeat with your left arm.

YIELD: 1 session

❓ **How it works:** Standing up and touching walls is a simple way to take a short, physical break and reset the brain. According to experts who study how to teach in ways that better match the way the brain learns, activities that cross the sides of your body—as in the arm and leg wraps and the infinity trace—stimulate and refresh the brain. Wrapping your arms and legs also stretches some muscles and temporarily constricts circulation. When you release, you feel a pleasant flush of fresh blood.

Essential Oil Lift

Peppermint essential oil

PREPARATION AND USE:

Place 5 to 10 drops of the oil on a cotton ball. Place the cotton in a clean jar and cap it. Whenever you need a boost, open the jar and sniff.

YIELD: Multiple sniffs

❓ How it works: A study showed that an inhaled mixture of peppermint, basil, helichrysum, and rose water reduced perceptions of mental exhaustion and burnout. Other essential oil candidates for countering fatigue include jasmine, basil, eucalyptus, lemon, rosemary, cardamom, cinnamon, cedarwood, cypress, and patchouli.

LIFESTYLE TIP

Chill on the caffeine. Caffeine can help you make it through to the day. But it doesn't make up for missed sleep. The effect of caffeine is similar to epinephrine (adrenaline). If you're stressed out, you already have enough of that hormone on board. Because it takes an average of five hours to break down half the caffeine in your bloodstream, afternoon consumption can interfere with much-needed sleep.

High Blood Pressure

It's dubbed the "silent killer" for good reason. This sneaky disease exhibits no signs or symptoms until significant damage is done. The first sign might be a heart attack or stroke—the leading causes of death in the United States. Some 65 million Americans have high blood pressure, or hypertension.

The rate is particularly high in African Americans. One study found that the rate of hypertension was nearly 48 percent in blacks versus 31 percent in whites. Furthermore, despite comparable treatment, blood pressure less often returned to normal in African Americans. Different ethnic groups may respond differently to blood pressure–lowering medications.

Blood pressure has two readings, measured in millimeters of mercury (abbreviated "mm Hg"). The top number reflects systolic pressure—the highest pressure, reached when the heart contracts. The bottom number reflects diastolic pressure—the lowest pressure just before the heart contracts again. Ideally, systolic pressure is lower than 120 mm Hg and diastolic pressure is lower than 80 mm Hg. Prehypertension is defined as a systolic blood pressure between 120 and 139 or diastolic blood pressure between 80 and 89 mm Hg. The threshold for hypertension starts at 140 systolic, 90 diastolic.

Hypertension damages arteries and taxes the heart. Pressure in the arteries comes from the force of the heart's contraction, the volume of blood, and the narrowness and stiffness of the arteries. With age, arteries lose elasticity. Atherosclerosis, a condition marked by fatty deposits in the arterial walls, can both cause and result from hypertension. Other consequences of hypertension can be heart disease, stroke, kidney damage, and vision-robbing eye disease.

Lifestyle changes can help lower blood pressure. They include reducing dietary salt, eating a plant-based diet, quitting smoking, exercising regularly, losing excess weight, and managing stress.

Doctors also prescribe medications: diuretics to increase loss of water in urine, beta blockers to slow the heart, and other medications aimed at dilating the arteries. If you're taking a prescription medication to lower blood pressure, do not stop—not without a discussion with your doctor. None of the following remedies is intended as a substitute for standard medical care.

Hibiscus Cooler

5 cups (1.2 L) water

½ cup (72 g) dried hibiscus calyces

1 cup (235 ml) pure pomegranate or cranberry juice

Juice of ½ lemon

PREPARATION AND USE:

Boil the water in a nonreactive (enamel or stainless-steel) pot. Remove from the heat. Add the dried hibiscus. Cover and steep for 15 minutes. Strain. Add the pomegranate and lemon juices. Drink warm or cold.

YIELD: 4 servings

❓ **How it works:** Studies show simply drinking tart, delicious hibiscus tea lowers blood pressure in people with prehypertension and moderate hypertension. One study found that hibiscus tea (consumed before breakfast for four weeks) compared favorably to the blood-pressure-lowering medication captopril. Regular consumption of hibiscus tea also lowers LDL cholesterol and triglycerides (blood fats) and raises HDL (good) cholesterol. Both pomegranate and cranberry can lower blood pressure. All of these plants are rich in antioxidant and cardiovascular-protecting plant compounds called flavonoids.

Note: Pomegranate juice is naturally sweet. If you use cranberry juice, which is very tart, add honey or agave nectar to taste. The calyx in hibiscus forms a cup under the petals. You can find dried hibiscus in bulk in some natural food stores and in Mexican food stores, where they may be sold as "flores de Jamaica."

Heart-Healthy Cocoa Smoothie

Incorporating small amounts of cocoa or dark chocolate into your daily diet can protect your heart and blood vessels.

1 large banana

1 cup (235 ml) almond milk

2 to 3 (10 to 15 g) tablespoons unsweetened cocoa powder

1 tablespoon (20 g) honey or agave

1 teaspoon (2 g) flaxseeds

PREPARATION AND USE:

Combine all the ingredients in a blender or food processor and blend until smooth. Enjoy!

YIELD: 1 to 2 servings

❓ How it works: Chocolate and cocoa power come from dried beans of the cacao tree. The flavonoids in chocolate and cocoa reduce blood pressure—the darker the chocolate, the higher the flavonoids. Cocoa powder also contains fiber, which can help curb cholesterol, as do the flax seeds.

Go Fish! Hors d'Oeuvre

In our household, when Dad opened a can of sardines, it was a special occasion. They were delicious doled out on simple saltines. Little did we know that we were keeping our blood pressure in check. ~ BBG

1 can (8- to 12-count) oil-packed sardines

12 to 16 whole-grain crackers

Lemon wedges

Sprigs of parsley

PREPARATION AND USE:

Spread each cracker with a half sardine. Squeeze lemon juice on top. Add parsley to garnish. Enjoy!

YIELD: 4 servings

❓ **How it works:** The omega-3 fatty acids in fish oil have been shown to reduce blood pressure in people with mild hypertension, mainly from fatty fish, such as mackerel and salmon. Sardines are at the top of the list.

Depressurizing Tonic

For an extra punch, Linda substitutes hibiscus tea for the liquid in this recipe.

2 teaspoons (10 ml) apple cider vinegar

1 cup (235 ml) water or pomegranate juice

PREPARATION AND USE:

Mix the vinegar and liquid. Drink the tonic once a day.

YIELD: 1 application

❓ **How it works:** Apple cider vinegar, an apple product, contains flavonoids. Apple cider vinegar has been used as a tonic for blood pressure and other ailments for centuries. Recent animal and preliminary human studies show that the flavonoid quercetin in apples may help lower blood pressure and improve heart health.

❗ **Warning:** Check with your doctor before using. Large doses of apple cider vinegar over a long period of time can burn the mouth and throat or erode tooth enamel; it may also counteract medications for heart and kidney disease.

Melonmania

In general, whole fruit contains fiber and phytochemicals that are just plain good for you. The potassium in melon helps control high blood pressure.

2 cups (340 g) seeded honeydew melon chunks

2 cups (300 g) watermelon chunks

PREPARATION AND USE:

Mix the fruit in a large bowl. Don't remove the seeds from the watermelon chunks. See why below.

YIELD: 2 to 4 servings

❓ **How it works:** All melons, especially honeydew, contain potassium. As noted earlier, reducing dietary intake of sodium and optimizing intake of potassium can help bring blood pressure under control. Eat your watermelon, seeds and all. The seeds of watermelon have a juice that contains L-citrulline, an amino acid the body converts to L-arginine, another amino acid, which relaxes arteries. A 2013 study in older women found that consumption of a watermelon supplement reduced arterial stiffness and blood pressure.

Purple Potato Salad

For the salad:

3 medium-size (or 6 small) purple potatoes, scrubbed thoroughly

2 large eggs

1 celery stalk, diced

½ onion, diced

1 tablespoon (4 g) crushed fresh dill

Pinch of freshly ground black pepper and paprika or cayenne, or your choice of other salt-free seasoning

For the dressing:

1 cup (230 g) plain low-fat yogurt

3 tablespoons (45 g) deli brown or honey mustard

1 packet (1 g) stevia

PREPARATION AND USE:

Place the potatoes and eggs in separate pots of water and bring both to a boil. Boil the potatoes for about 20 minutes until tender. Bring the eggs to a boil, then remove from the heat, cover, and set aside for 10 to 12 minutes. Let cool. Cut the potatoes, including their skin, into bite-size chunks and place in a medium-size bowl. Peel, dice, and add the egg whites (toss the cholesterol-rich yolk). Add the celery, onion, dill, and seasonings. In a separate bowl, mix together the yogurt, mustard, and stevia. Fold into the salad and serve.

YIELD: 4 servings

❓ **How it works:** These spuds have high levels of chlorogenic acid, shown to reduce blood pressure. And they're antioxidant-rich—one key to reducing inflammation that causes heart disease.

Immune System Support

Microorganisms are everywhere—in the air, soil, and water. Humans are like small planets colonized by billions of bacteria and fungi. The bacteria carpeting our intestinal tract alone outnumber our own cells by a factor of ten. Fortunately, most of these tiny denizens benefit us by manufacturing vitamins, outcompeting disease-causing microbes, and otherwise contributing to immune function.

Nevertheless, a large number of microbes—viruses, bacteria, fungi, protozoa, and worms—can make us sick. So if they're everywhere, why aren't we sick all the time? You guessed it: the immune system. This complex association of organs, cells, and molecules protects us from anything foreign and potentially harmful: "bad" microbes, cancer cells, splinters, toxic chemicals. Ideally, it refrains from attacking harmless pollen, animal dander, and our normal cells. But allergies and autoimmune diseases do occur.

Certain people have more trouble maintaining a healthy immune system than others. Elderly people often have diminished immune defense. Chronic sleep deprivation causes imbalances in the immune system and results in increased inflammation. Chronic stress overload dampens immune system function. Certain medications (corticosteroids and chemotherapy) and procedures (radiation therapy) suppress the immune system. Surgical procedures stress the body and also raise the risk for infection. Finally, some diseases either present at birth or acquired later (AIDS, mononucleosis, leukemia, and diabetes) impair the immune system. Fortunately, a host of simple lifestyle choices and a few nutritional supplements can ironclad your immune system. Key among them is taking care of yourself. Undue stress, sleep deprivation, a diet of processed foods high in sugar and fat, social isolation, and inactivity undermine general health and the immune system.

Pumpkin Pleasure Soup

3½ cups (406 g) fresh pumpkin, or 2 cans (15 ounces, or 528 g)
   pure pumpkin purée (if pumpkin is not in season)
Enough water to just cover the fresh pumpkin, if used
2½ cups (570 ml) low-fat coconut milk
1 teaspoon (6 g) salt
½ teaspoon ground nutmeg
½ teaspoon ground allspice
Freshly ground black pepper

PREPARATION AND USE:

Cut the pumpkin into chunks and place in a large pan. Barely cover the
pumpkin with water. Bring to a boil. Lower the heat and simmer for about
20 minutes. Puree the pumpkin, using a stand or immersion blender, and
keep it warm. (Alternatively, place the canned pumpkin in a large pan
without water and heat.) Stir in the coconut milk, salt, nutmeg, allspice, and
pepper to taste. Serve warm.

YIELD: About 4 servings

❓ **How it works:** Pumpkin is rich in carotenoids, which neutralize free
radicals and support immune health. Our bodies convert some of these
carotenoids to vitamin A, which is also critical for proper immune function.
Many spices are antibacterial, including cinnamon, nutmeg, and allspice.

Medicinal Mushroom Sauté

Maitake is Japanese for "dancing mushroom." Perhaps people danced for joy upon finding this treasure (also called hen of the woods) in the wild.

1½ teaspoons (8 ml) olive oil

2 teaspoons (10 g) butter

1½ teaspoons (8 ml) balsamic vinegar

1 pound (455 g) fresh maitake mushrooms

1 garlic clove, minced

PREPARATION AND USE:

Place the oil and butter in a large skillet and melt over medium heat. Stir in the balsamic vinegar. Add the mushrooms. Sauté for about 15 minutes or until tender. Add the garlic at the end of the cooking time and sauté for about a minute: active ingredients in garlic do not survive prolonged cooking. Sprinkle the mushrooms over a bed of wilted spinach for a delicious salad, fold them into an omelet, or enjoy them alone, as a side dish.

YIELD: 4 to 6 servings

❓ How it works: Maitake mushrooms, along with shiitake, are among the top medicinal mushrooms. Shiitake has antiviral, anticancer molecules called interferons. Studies show complex polysaccharides from the maitake mushroom enhance immune function and also have anticancer effects. Recipe Variation: Substitute shiitake mushrooms for maitake mushrooms, which are harder to find fresh, or make a mix. If you use dried mushrooms, 3 ounces (85 g, about ⅓ cup) will substitute for a pound (455 g) of fresh. First, reconstitute by soaking in boiling-hot water for 20 minutes (save the water for soup stock).

Immune Soup

Years ago, herbalist and author Brigitte Mars told me about this recipe.
Since then, I've adapted the recipe and make it at the first sign a family
member has a cold. ~ LBW

2 tablespoons (30 ml) olive oil

1 large onion, chopped

2 chicken breasts (skin removed), or 1 pound (455 g) extra-firm tofu

1 quart (946 ml) vegetable or chicken stock

1 quart (946 ml) water

4 to 6 fresh shiitake mushrooms, or 8 to 10 dried

1 cup (100 g) chopped celery,

2 cups (260 g) chopped carrots or other

root vegetables

4 to 5 astragalus roots

2 teaspoons (2.8 g) dried thyme

1 teaspoon (1. g) dried rosemary

1 teaspoon (1 g) dried oregano

½ teaspoon dried sage

4 garlic cloves, minced

2 tablespoons (8 g) chopped fresh parsley

Cracked pepper (optional)

PREPARATION AND USE:

In a large stockpot, heat the olive oil over medium heat. Add the onion
and sauté until soft, 3 to 5 minutes. If using chicken, sauté it, too, adding
¼ cup (60 ml) of the stock or water to keep it from sticking. Once the
chicken is cooked through, 7 to 10 minutes on each side, remove it from
the pot, cube it, and place it in the refrigerator. In the same pan, sauté the

mushrooms over medium heat until gently browned, 3 to 5 minutes. Add the remaining stock and the remaining water. Bring to a boil. Add the remaining vegetables and astragalus roots. Lower the heat, cover, and simmer for 30 minutes. Add the tofu now (if you're using it rather than chicken) and the thyme, rosemary, oregano, and sage. Simmer for another 20 minutes or until the vegetables are tender. Return the chicken to the pot and heat over low heat another 5 minutes. (You should have enough liquid to generously cover all the vegetables. If not, add more water.)

Turn off the heat. Fish out the astragalus roots, which are too fibrous to eat. Add the garlic, parsley, and, if desired, cracked pepper to taste. Serve.

YIELD: 4 hearty servings

? **How it works:** Shiitake mushrooms, garlic, and onions all enhance immune function. Garlic and onion are also antimicrobial. If you can't find shiitake mushrooms, all mushrooms contain complicated polysaccharides called beta-glucans, which enhance immune system function. Astragalus root also contains polysaccharides and other chemicals that support the immune system. You may find the dried roots (which look like tongue depressors) in the bulk section at your natural food store or order them online. Chinese medicine doctors use extracts of this root to enhance immune function in people being treated for cancer (radiation and chemotherapy often suppress immune function). Studies support that use. Rosemary, thyme, and oregano all carry antimicrobial action.

Recipe Variations: Feel free to experiment with the seasonings. You can, for instance, use curry spices instead of Italian seasonings. Rather than using vegetable or chicken stock, you can blend 2 tablespoons (32 g) of white miso paste with 1 quart (946 ml) of hot water.

Nut Pick-Me-Up

We love this recipe for parties—little do the guests suspect they are consuming nutrients that support the immune system.

½ cup (75 g) unsalted peanuts

½ cup (73 g) unsalted almonds

¼ cup unsalted (36 g) sunflower seeds

1 teaspoon (5 ml) olive oil

1 teaspoon (6 g) sea salt

PREPARATION AND USE:

Preheat the oven to 350°F (180°C, or gas mark 4). Mix the nuts with the olive oil. Spread across a baking sheet. Bake for about 10 minutes. Remove from the oven and sprinkle with the salt. Let cool for an hour before serving. Pop a handful into your mouth.

YIELD: Five ¼-cup (38 g) servings

❓ How it works: Peanuts, almonds, and sunflower seeds are rich in zinc and vitamin E. The immune system needs vitamin E as an antioxidant and to manufacture important regulatory molecules. Low zinc intake impairs immune function. If you take supplements, take care not to overdo it. The recommended intake is 11 milligrams for men and 8 milligrams for women (11 milligrams for pregnant women).Too much zinc from supplements can cause problems. But you can't go wrong with eating zinc-rich foods, including oysters, crab, wheat germ, and pumpkin and squash seeds.

Circulation-Boosting Salt Scrub

This scrub leaves skin feeling toned and silky while enhancing blood circulation for a healthier, livelier you.

1 cup (240 g) sea salt (avoid regular table salt, which is harsh on skin)

½ cup (120 ml) olive oil

5 drops peppermint oil

PREPARATION AND USE:

Put the salt in a small bowl. Mix in the olive oil so that mixture is moist and holds together but is not overly oily. Drop in the peppermint oil, blending with each drop. Soften your skin by soaking in a tub for 10 minutes. Drain the tub, pat yourself dry, and sit on the side of the tub. Apply a small amount of the scrub to each leg. With a warm, moist washcloth, slowly scrub each leg, not rubbing too hard and moving upward, toward your heart. Repeat with your arms and torso, always toward your heart. Rinse off in a warm shower. Finish with a burst of cold water.

YIELD: 3 to 4 applications

? How it works: Massaging in salt and essential oils increases blood circulation. Warm water dilates blood vessels (making you look pink). The quick burst of cold water at the end constricts blood vessels. The total effect is immediate invigoration, cleansing, and ultimate relaxation.

Note: The oil creates a slippery surface, so step carefully.

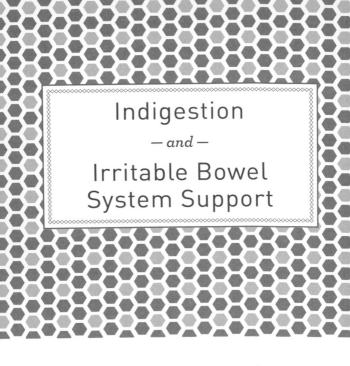

Indigestion

— and —

Irritable Bowel System Support

Everyone has an Achilles' heel. For many Americans, the weak point is the gut. It may not take much—a change in diet, some added stress—to create gastrointestinal (GI) distress. For some people, the symptoms are felt in the upper part of the GI system; for others, the lower GI system generates discomfort.

Dyspepsia is another term for indigestion. Symptoms, which originate from the stomach and first part of the small intestine, include pain or burning high in the abdomen (below the tip of the breastbone), early satiety (feeling full after a few bites), feeling heaviness after eating, and belching. For many people, symptoms coincide with mealtimes. Likewise, lower GI symptoms are often associated with meals. They can include gas, bloating, and cramping. In a condition called irritable bowel syndrome (IBS), additional symptoms include diarrhea and/or constipation.

Dyspepsia and irritable bowel syndrome fall into the category of "functional" rather than "organic" disorders. In the former, the problem lies with the performance of the system, but without visible signs of disease. In organic disorders, there is a visible lesion such an ulcer. Examples include peptic ulcers and inflammatory bowel diseases.

The potential causes of functional bowel conditions are multiple. They include stress overload; hypersensitivity of intestinal nerves; imbalances in the bacterial ecology of the intestines; food allergies and intolerances; medications, such as nonsteroidal anti-inflammatory drugs and antibiotics; and chronic diseases, such as hypothyroidism, diabetes, anxiety, and depression.

Light Your Fire Salad

Traditional Chinese medicine practitioners speak of "digestive fire." If you experience burning sensations with meals, don't let this description alarm you. It refers to stimulating enzymes to better digest your food.

1 cup (20 g) torn arugula

1 cup (50 g) torn endive

1 cup (40 g) torn radicchio

2 tablespoons (30 ml) balsamic vinegar

1 garlic clove, minced

Freshly ground black pepper, to taste

¼ cup (60 ml) olive oil

¼ cup (20 g) shaved Parmesan cheese

PREPARATION AND USE:

Toss together the greens in a large bowl and set aside. Pour the vinegar into a large salad bowl. Add the garlic and few sprinkles of pepper. Drizzle the olive oil into the bowl, stirring briskly with a whisk until the mixture is light brown. Empty the bowl of greens into the salad bowl with dressing. Toss. Sprinkle with the Parmesan shavings and serve immediately.

YIELD: 4 to 6 servings

? How it works: Herbalists have long used digestive bitters, drunk before the meal, to jump-start digestion. A European tradition is eating a salad of bitter greens after the main meal. Bitters stimulate bile and digestive enzymes.

Mango Summer Aperitif

This elegant yet easy aperitif stimulates your appetite and prepares your digestive system for a meal. Aperitif comes from the Latin verb aperire, "to open."

2 cups (350 g) mango chunks, frozen
½ cup (120 ml) Muscat or Dolce dessert wine
1 bottle (750 ml) dry champagne, chilled

PREPARATION AND USE:

Partially thaw the mango chunks. Blend the mango in blender. Add the dessert wine and blend slightly. Fill champagne flutes half-full with the mango mixture. Top with chilled champagne and serve.

YIELD: 6 servings

? **How it works:** Dry champagne stimulates digestion. In addition to being rich in essential nutrients, mango contains fiber, which promotes healthy intestinal microbes and regular bowel movements.

Note: Alcohol aggravates heartburn. If you have this condition, consider substituting pomegranate juice for the alcohol.

Après-Dinner Digestif

In France, a digestif, often brandy or a liqueur, is sipped after meals to aid digestion. You can make your own, with digestion-aiding fennel.

2 tablespoons (12 g) fennel seeds

½ cup (50 g) fresh, chopped fennel stalks and leaves

1½ cups (355 ml) vodka

Honey

PREPARATION AND USE:

Put the fennel seeds, stalks, and leaves into a clean pint-size (475 ml) jar. Pour the vodka over the plant matter until you have a good 2 inches (5 cm) of alcohol above the top of the fennel. Cap and shake well. Place in a cupboard for one to two weeks, shaking occasionally.

When ready, place a strainer over a small mixing bowl. Lay a square of cheesecloth over the strainer, with about an inch (2.5 cm) of extra material hanging over the sides of the strainer. Carefully pour the contents of the jar through the cheesecloth.

Use a spoon to scoop out all the fennel onto the cheesecloth. With clean hands, gather the edges of the cheesecloth. Squeeze out as much of the liquid as you can into the bowl. Remove the strainer. Discard the spent fennel.

Measure the amount of liquid. To that amount, add half as much honey. (For instance, if you have 1 cup [235 ml] of fennel extract, stir ½ cup [160 ml] of honey into it.) Wash and dry the jar and pour your digestif into it. Store in the refrigerator or in the freezer for a cold, refreshing drink. After dinner, pour 1 ounce (28 ml) of the drink into a small digestif glass and sip. You may also dilute it with 1 tablespoon (15 ml) of water.

YIELD: Multiple small servings

How it works: Fennel is in the parsley family, along with carrots, celery, anise, caraway, and licorice. All have value for the digestive tract. Fennel is a carminative herb, meaning it helps expel gas from the stomach and intestines. It's also traditionally used to relieve nausea and vomiting, inflammation, and intestinal spasms.

Note: An herbal extract with alcohol and water (and vodka contains a good balance of the two) is called a tincture. The addition of honey creates a liqueur that's sweet enough to enjoy in small amounts without cutting it with water. Feel free to try to the recipe without honey. If you do, we recommend diluting it with water before consuming.

After-Dinner Digestive Snack

1 tablespoon (6 g) aniseeds
1 tablespoon (6 g) fennel seeds

PREPARATION AND USE:

Put the seeds into a small, clean jar, cap, and shake to mix. After dinner, put ¼ teaspoon of the seed mixture into the palm of your hand and pop into your mouth. Savor the taste as you chew.

YIELD: 24 servings

❓ **How it works:** See the explanation in the previous recipe for fennel. Also a member of the parsley family, anise has similar properties to fennel. It relieves bloating, flatulence, nausea, cramping, and poor appetite. Both seeds also freshen the breath.

Warming Digestive Tea

These herbs and spices are both sweet and slightly bitter to improve digestion.

1 tablespoon (2 g) dried peppermint leaves

1 teaspoon (2 g) fennel seeds

1 teaspoon (2 g) aniseeds

1 teaspoon (5 g) cinnamon chips, from a crushed cinnamon stick

½ teaspoon cardamom seeds

2 cups (475 ml) water

PREPARATION AND USE:

Combine the peppermint and spices in a clean jar. Boil the water in a saucepan. Add the spice mixture. Cover and steep for 15 minutes. Strain and enjoy before and after meals.

YIELD: 2 servings

❓ **How it works:** See previous descriptions of anise and fennel. Cardamom also relieves intestinal spasms, gas, bloating, and flatulence. Peppermint relieves pain, cramping, and gas. Studies show that encapsulated peppermint oil significantly reduces symptoms of irritable bowel syndrome and dyspepsia.

A Digestive "New Leaf"

1 artichoke

Pinch of salt

1 teaspoon (5 ml) fresh lemon juice

1 tablespoon (15 ml) olive oil

1 teaspoon (3 g) minced fresh garlic

PREPARATION AND USE:

Slice off the artichoke top, trim the thorny tips and stem, and place in a steamer basket. In a pot, place about 2 inches (5 cm) of water, the salt, and the lemon juice and bring to a boil. Steam the artichoke in the pot, covered, for about 30 minutes (until the bottom of the artichoke can be pierced). In a clean bowl, stir together the olive oil and garlic. Remove the artichoke from the pot and allow it to cool. Pull off each artichoke petal and dip it into the olive oil mixture. Enjoy pulling the flesh off the base of the petal with your teeth. When all the petals are pulled away, scoop out and discard the fuzzy center. The fleshy artichoke heart remains. Slice it and enjoy on a salad or just plain. Many think it's the best part.

YIELD: 1 serving or 2, if cut in half

❓ **How it works:** Artichoke, a botanical relative of milk thistle, is the main ingredient in the Italian bitter aperitif Cynar. Milk thistle seeds are a bitter digestive tonic and also protect the liver and stimulate it to make bile. The seeds are one ingredient in a botanical formula shown to reduce symptoms of irritable bowel syndrome and dyspepsia. Although artichoke hasn't been as well researched, studies have shown that leaf extracts also significantly reduce dyspepsia and irritable bowel syndrome.

Umeboshi Snack

Umeboshi is a salty, pickled Japanese plum. The taste is tart and zingy.

1 cucumber

Umeboshi paste (see note)

1 teaspoon (3 g) sesame seeds, toasted

PREPARATION AND USE:

Wash and slice the cucumber into sturdy rounds, leaving the skin on. Add
a very thin layer of umeboshi paste to each cucumber slice. (The taste is
tangy and refreshing: a little goes a long way.) Sprinkle with sesame seeds.
Serve this quick and refreshing snack between meals or as an appetizer.

YIELD: 8 appetizer servings

❓ How it works: Umeboshi stimulates digestion, starting with increased
salivation. The fiber in sunflower seeds contributes to overall bowel health.
Soluble fiber inside the cucumber peel helps with digestive problems if you
have constipation. Peel the cucumber if it causes you to have gas or diarrhea.

Note: You can buy umeboshi paste in a local Asian food store.

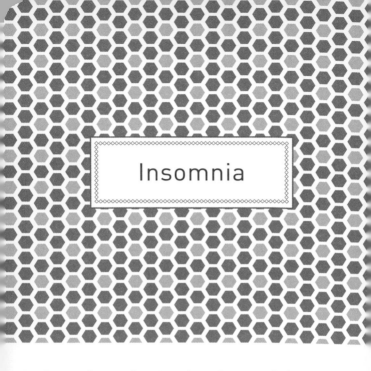

Insomnia

"To sleep, perchance to dream." Hamlet's reflection was for him, and for millions of Americans, wishful thinking. At any one time, up to a quarter of the population has insomnia, defined as an inability to fall and/or stay asleep. Nearly everyone has had at least one fretful night. Unfortunately, 10 percent of adults have chronic insomnia. For a variety of reasons, women are more often troubled with insomnia than are men.

Chronic insomnia erodes quality of life. Compared to their rested peers, people who don't get enough sleep are at risk for accidents (including car crashes and falls), infections, depression, weight problems, high blood pressure, heart disease, and diabetes. Poor concentration and thinking skills erode productivity. Tired people miss more work and decline social engagements. The personal and societal impact is enormous.

Ideally, treatment resolves the underlying problem that keeps the person awake: psychological stress, anxiety, depression, heartburn, chronic cough, night sweats associated with menopause, frequent urination in older men with enlarged prostates, sleep disorders, and more. Sometimes all that's needed is to improve what's called "sleep hygiene." That means you use your bed only for sleep and sex. In addition:

- Don't do any of the following in bed: pay bills, argue, do homework, or watch television. It's also a good idea not to do mentally stimulating things just before bed, either.
- Create soothing bedtime rituals.
- Find time for physical activity each day, but avoid vigorous exercise just before bed. Stretching is fine.
- Go to bed and arise at more or less the same time every day. Most people need about 8 hours of sleep a night. (And your brain keeps track of any accumulating debt.) Give yourself a cushion of 30 minutes for falling asleep.
- Make your bedroom a warm, dark, inviting place. Even low light can disrupt melatonin, a hormone that regulates sleep and other rhythms. Cover glowing LED lights with a cloth. Turn your alarm clock to face the wall.
- Banish self-defeating thoughts. The problem with chronic insomnia is a dread of bedtime. Welcome it. Each night is a fresh start.

Lavender Bath Bomb

1 cup (221 g) baking soda

½ cup (65 g) cornstarch

½ cup (120 g) Epsom salts

½ cup (197 g) powdered citric acid

1 tablespoon (15 ml) water

2 teaspoons (10 ml) lavender essential oil

1 tablespoon (15 ml) melted coconut oil or vegetable oil

PREPARATION AND USE:

In a large glass bowl, combine all the dry ingredients. Whisk until smooth. In a separate small glass bowl, mix together the liquids (they will not blend perfectly). While continuing to whisk the dry ingredients, slowly add the liquid, about 1 teaspoon (5 ml) at a time—do not add too quickly or the ingredients will react. The final consistency should be like damp (not wet) sand and should hold together in a clump. If too dry, add another teaspoon (5 ml) of oil mixed with a teaspoon (5 ml) of water. If too wet, add small amounts of cornstarch. Press into muffin tins, filling halfway. Once dry, pop out the bombs and store in a tightly capped jar. Add one bomb to a warm bath and soothe away.

YIELD: 8 to 12 bombs, depending on the size of your mold

❓ **How it works:** The warmth of the bath soothes and relaxes. The Epsom salts relax the muscles. The lavender is calming.

Lavender Foot Massage

1 ounce (28 g) carrier oil (e.g., almond, apricot, grape seed, jojoba, or olive oil)

12 drops lavender essential oil (6 drops for pregnant women and children)

PREPARATION AND USE:

Pour the oil and lavender essential oil into a clean jar. Cap and shake. Wash and dry your feet. Sitting comfortably, draw a foot into your lap. Pour a palmful (about 1 tablespoon [15 ml]) of scented oil into your palm and massage into your foot. Take your time. Switch feet. If it's a chilly night, put on clean socks. Crawl into bed.

YIELD: 1 application

❓ How it works: Lavender is calming. The essential oil crosses the skin to enter the blood. It also enters via the lungs when you inhale the aroma. Massaging your feet literally takes you out of your busy head to help you settle down for the night. A 2013 study found inhalation of a blend of calming essential oils (lavender, Roman chamomile, and neroli) lowered anxiety and improved sleep quality in cardiac patients in the intensive care unit (a place notorious for disrupting sleep). You don't have to be sick to get the benefits. A study in healthy Japanese students showed that nighttime inhalation of lavender made them feel more refreshed come morning.

Variation: Ask a friend or partner to rub your feet (or back) for you. Feel free to experiment with other calming essential oils, such as Roman chamomile, bergamot, rose geranium, melissa (lemon balm), neroli, jasmine, ylang ylang, and sandalwood. What's important is whether you find the aroma relaxing.

Milk It!

1 cup (235 ml) milk

Honey or stevia

1 cardamom seed or 1 clove, crushed

PREPARATION AND USE:

Heat the milk with the cardamom in a small pan. Bring to a boil and then lower the heat to low. Simmer for 3 minutes. Add honey or stevia to taste. Simmer for 1 minute more. Remove from the heat and cover. Set aside for 5 minutes. Strain. Drink the warm milk before going to bed.

YIELD: 1 serving

? How it works: A cup of warm milk has long been revered as a sleep aid. It was once thought that milk's tryptophan (an amino acid that forms the backbone to the brain chemical serotonin and the hormone melatonin, both of which influence sleep) was the key ingredient. However, more recent studies suggest that commercially sold milk doesn't really improve sleep. Scientists hold that warm milk before bed is simply soothing—even if it's all in your head. Cardamom has been traditionally used to settle the digestive system.

Total Body Scrunch

You

Your bed

PREPARATION AND USE:

Lie on your bed. Draw your tailbone down to protect your low back. Lift your arms and legs (the Superman pose). Release. Roll onto your back again, pull your whole body into a ball, knees to chest, arms wrapped around legs. Scrunch your face and pull it toward your knees. Release back onto the bed. Let go. Really let go. Feel how warm and relaxed your muscles are. Feel the way the mattress and pillow support you. If you awaken in the night, repeat this exercise out of bed, if you're sharing space with a partner.

YIELD: 1 session

❓ **How it works:** Complete muscle exertion helps you fully relax, bringing you closer to sleep. In the evening, light yoga or stretches can also help bring you closer to sleep. With practice, you can lie down, do a mental body scan, and quickly release any identified areas of tension.

Sleepy-Time Quick Flex

You

Your bed (or a soft pad or rug)

PREPARATION AND USE:

Lie on your back. Sequentially tighten and release every muscle in your body: hands | arms | feet | legs | buttocks | stomach | neck

Scrunch your face. Open your eyes wide and stick out your tongue as far as you can. Now totally relax. Sink into the mattress and pillow. Repeat if you awaken in the middle of the night.

YIELD: 1 session

❓ **How it works:** Progressive muscle tightening and relaxation helps you focus on how warm and heavy the muscles feel, making you drowsy. Repeat this all the way up your body, ending at your neck and face. When you finish you should feel quieter physically and mentally.

Count Your Breaths

You

A quiet place

PREPARATION AND USE:

Breathe in, making the inhalation as long and as slow as you can. Count silently. It doesn't matter whether you count slowly (one-one thousand, two-one thousand) to four or to ten. Exhale as long and as slowly as you can, again counting silently. Repeat until you relax and feel sleepy.

YIELD: 1 session

? How it works: Similar to counting sheep, this exercise makes it hard to think about other things, so you begin to relax. The slow breaths calm your nervous system. Studies show that, even in people with serious medical conditions, the breath work used in yoga (plus or minus yoga poses) improves sleep quality.

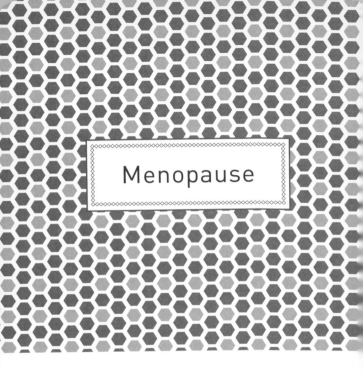

Menopause

Menopause is like climate change writ small. The woman's climate becomes more tropical, but at somewhat unpredictable moments. Like global warming, menopause can be inconvenient, such as when you're standing before a group of college students and have to stop mid-lecture to pare down to your camisole.

In menopause, the ovaries shut down for business. Estrogen and progesterone fall dramatically. Menstrual periods cease. (Yes, there is good news. That, and the hair on your arms and legs thins—seemingly by migrating to your chin.)

The average age of natural menopause is fifty-one. The long warm-up period is called perimenopause. It can last for years. Progesterone often wanes before estrogen, which can lead to more frequent, heavier periods. Some women also notice mood swings and more frequent headaches. As estrogen levels plummet, hot flashes occur. Night sweats and other menopause-related changes can interrupt sleep. Concentration may waver. Vaginal tissues become thinner and drier. Sex drive can decline—though some of that is psychological (whether you find yourself and your mate attractive). The skin, mouth, and eyes may also become drier. Some women breeze through perimenopause to menopause; others suffer.

For years, conventional treatment has focused on hormone replacement therapy (HRT)—the name for the combined use of estrogen and progesterone. Women at risk for breast cancer can't use any kind of HRT. Alternative prescription medications can help. So can lifestyle changes, such as incorporating breathable materials (e.g., a mattress pad without the rubberized backing or wearing cotton nightclothes) to combat sleep-interrupting night sweats.

Artery-Enhancing Olive Oil Dressing

Menopausal women are at greater risk for heart disease. Keep your heart tuned up with this healthy dressing.

¼ cup (60 ml) extra-virgin olive oil

¼ cup (60 ml) red wine vinegar

¾ teaspoon dried oregano

¼ teaspoon salt substitute

Pinch of freshly ground black pepper

PREPARATION AND USE:

Combine all the ingredients in a blender and blend. Pour over salads rich in leafy green vegetables.

YIELD: ⅓ cup (80 ml) dressing (refrigerate leftovers)

❓ **How it works:** Extra-virgin olive oil, which is good for the heart and arteries, helps menopausal women guard against cardiovascular disease. Leafy greens in salads provide calcium and other nutrients to help stave off bone loss. Plus, filling up on lightly dressed salads (rather than, say, French fries) can help stave off the weight creep that often affects women past menopause.

Leafy Greens and Tofu Sauté

2 cups (72 g) Swiss chard

2 cups (60 g) baby spinach, rinsed and drained

2 cups (40 g) arugula

2 cups (134 g) kale

1 tablespoon (15 ml) vegetable oil

1 block (14 ounces, or 400 g) firm tofu, cut into 1-inch (2.5 cm) chunks

1 garlic clove, minced

¼ cup (30 g) walnut halves and pieces

¼ cup (35 g) raisins or (30 g) dried cranberries

PREPARATION AND USE:

Tear the greens into small pieces. Heat the oil in a large skillet or wok over medium heat. Add the tofu and sauté for about 5 minutes. Add the garlic and sauté for about a minute. Increase the heat to medium-high and add the greens. Stir with a wooden spoon until wilted. Reduce the heat to low and add 1 teaspoon (5 ml) water. Cover and allow to steam for 3 minutes. Mix in the walnuts and raisins and serve.

YIELD: 4 servings

❓ **How it works:** Tofu, made of soybeans, contains isoflavones (plant substances that act as phytoestrogens—they stimulate estrogen receptors). Research indicates that consuming soy protein (20 to 60 grams a day, which provides 34 to 76 milligrams of isoflavones) can reduce hot flashes. Also, soy, leafy dark greens, and walnuts are rich in bone-friendly minerals, such as calcium and magnesium, which may slow bone loss after menopause.

Tea for Sage Women

This earthy and pungent tea can help ground women as menopause takes flight.

2 cups (475 ml) water

1 tablespoon (2 g) crumbled dry sage leaves, or 2 tablespoons (5 g) chopped fresh

Honey (optional)

PREPARATION AND USE:

Boil the water. Turn off the heat and add the sage. Cover and steep for 10 minutes. Strain. Add honey, if desired, to taste.

YIELD: 1 large serving or 2 small servings

❓ **How it works:** Sage is a traditional remedy for excessive perspiration. It also contains a chemical called geraniol that acts as a phytoestrogen. A 2011 Swiss study showed that a fresh sage extract taken for eight weeks significantly reduced hot flashes and associated menopausal symptoms relative to placebo.

❗ **Warning:** Limit to three cups a day. Sage comes in a couple species: common garden sage (*Salvia officinalis*) and Spanish sage (*Salvia lavandulaefolia*). The former contains thujone, a chemical that, in higher doses, can be toxic to the nervous system and stimulate seizures in vulnerable people. Aside from use as a food seasoning, pregnant and nursing women should avoid medicinal doses of garden sage (as it can stimulate uterine contractions and bleeding and also diminish breast milk).

Savory and Grounding Lentil Soup

This soup is rich and soothing and delicious with a loaf of French bread. It refrigerates well so you can enjoy it for several days.

1½ cups (288 g) dried lentils

2 tablespoons (28 ml) vegetable oil

1 onion, diced

3 garlic cloves, minced

1 can (14.5 ounces, or 411 g) diced tomatoes

2 carrots, peeled and diced

2 celery stalks, diced

1 quart (946 ml) vegetable stock

2 sage leaves, or 1 teaspoon (1 g) dried sage

2 bay leaves

½ teaspoon ground cumin

Sea salt and freshly ground black pepper

PREPARATION AND USE:

Rinse the lentils and then soak them in water for at least 1 hour. Pour the oil into a large saucepan over medium heat. Sauté the onion and garlic for about 2 minutes. Add the tomatoes, carrots, and celery and sauté for 3 to 5 minutes more. Pour in the stock and add the sage, bay leaves, cumin, and salt and pepper to taste. Stir in the lentils and bring to a boil. Lower the heat to low and simmer for 20 minutes. Remove the bay and sage leaves before serving.

YIELD: 6 servings

❓ **How it works:** Legumes other than soy contain phytoestrogens. Soy just happens to have the highest content and the most research study.

Salad Pepper-Uppers

We love the crunchy pick-me-up these seeds add to a salad.

Handful of pomegranate arils or sesame seeds

PREPARATION AND USE:

Sprinkle the arils or seeds over salads or soups.

YIELD: 1 serving

🛈 **How it works:** Both pomegranate arils and sesame seeds have phytoestrogens, the chemical that makes soy a menopausal favorite. A 2012 study showed mild benefits for a pomegranate seed oil taken for twelve weeks (though the effects didn't reach the threshold for statistical significance in reducing hot flashes and other menopausal symptoms). The authors called for further studies on pomegranate. Pomegranate does contain a number of healthful nutrients, flavonoids, and omega-3 fatty acids.

Yoga Stretch

This flowing exercise stretches your entire body, wakes up your spine, and calms and focuses your brain.

You

Loose, stretchable clothing or yoga wear

A floor or flat ground

PREPARATION AND USE:

Stand with both feet planted on the ground, about hip distance apart. Distribute your weight evenly on your feet (front to back, side to side). Extend your arms at your sides, fingertips pointing down. Align the back of your head and shoulders over your heels. Feel your shoulder blades slide down your back. Raise your arms over your head on an inhalation. Pause. Holding your core muscles steady, exhale as you slowly swan dive forward. If your fingertips don't touch your toes, bend your knees. Inhaling, put your palms on your shins. Straighten your arms so that your back makes a table-top (with torso at a 90-degree angle to your legs). Exhaling, reach again toward your toes. Let your head and neck go. On an inhale, core solid, lift your arms and your torso back to standing (arms over head). Exhaling, bring your palms together in front of your heart. Close your eyes and breathe. Notice a difference?

YIELD: 1 stretch

? How it works: Recent studies show that yoga reduces some menopausal symptoms, though it may be more beneficial for associated psychological complaints and insomnia than hot flashes. If you haven't tried it, check to see whether beginner's yoga classes are offered in your neighborhood.

Morning Sickness

Nausea and vomiting are one of the most common complaints during a woman's pregnancy—and perhaps the first time that cracks appear in her romantic notions of motherhood. In fact, 50 to 90 percent of women have queasiness during the first trimester (the first thirteen weeks). Symptoms usually begin at the end of the first month, peak during the third month, and dissipate by week 14. Of all the races, white women are most commonly affected.

Up to 3 percent of women develop severe and persistent nausea and vomiting. This condition, called hyperemesis gravidarum, may require hospitalization to maintain nutrition and hydration. A number of factors are thought to cause nausea and vomiting in pregnancy. They include hormonal shifts, heightened sense of smell, psychological challenges, and genetics.

Fortunately, most women have mild symptoms. Although those symptoms may be miserable for you, the good news is that nausea and vomiting during pregnancy doesn't stunt your fetus's growth.

RECIPES TO TREAT MORNING SICKNESS

Morning Bedside Snack

Rice cakes, crackers, or dry toast

Peanut, cashew, or almond butter, or tahini

Glass of water

PREPARATION AND USE:

Prepare your snack the night before. (Or ask your partner to serve you in bed.) Spread the nut butter on the cakes or crackers and leave them on a plate at your bedside. (If nut butters suddenly seem loathsome, leave them off.) Before you do as much as lift your head from the pillow, nibble your snack. Sip the water. Take your time. Get up slowly.

YIELD: 1 snack

? How it works: Low blood sugar often triggers nausea and vomiting during pregnancy. Your goal is to prevent low blood sugar. Carbohydrates, especially refined carbohydrates, quickly raise blood sugar. While you sleep, you're fasting. That's why you want to break that fast as soon as possible. Try to eat a small meal every 2 hours.

B6 Boost

1 cup (30 g) spinach, rinsed and drained

¼ cup (56 g) diced, boiled potato

1 tablespoon (15 ml) olive oil

1 tablespoon (15 ml) balsamic vinegar

¼ cup (36 g) sunflower seeds

1 can (6 ounces, or 168 g) tuna or 6 ounces
(170 g) cooked chicken breast (optional)

1 hard-boiled large egg, sliced

1 slice whole wheat bread, toasted

PREPARATION AND USE:

Toss the spinach and potato in a salad bowl. Whisk the oil and vinegar in a
small bowl. Drizzle the vinaigrette into the salad and toss again. Toss in the
sunflower seeds. If the smell of tuna or chicken doesn't make you gag, add as
much as you want. Top with slices of egg. Nibble the toast as you eat the salad.

YIELD: 1 serving

❓ **How it works:** Several studies have shown that vitamin B6 supplements
reduce nausea in pregnancy. Spinach, sunflower seeds, potatoes, tuna,
chicken, and whole grains are all good sources of B6. Other sources include
nuts, peas, and beans. Eggs offer high protein, which takes longer to digest,
so it stays in your system longer. All of these foods contain
valuable nutrients.

Note: Use additional oil and vinegar, if desired, but keep their ratio 1:1.

Veggified Rice with Garlic and Ginger

1¾ cups (410 ml) water

1 garlic clove, minced

Pinch of salt

¾ cup (143 g) uncooked brown rice

1 broccoli floret, sliced

1 carrot, diced

½ red bell pepper, seeded and diced

½ onion, diced

½ teaspoon fresh minced fresh ginger

PREPARATION AND USE:

Add the garlic and salt to the water and bring to a boil. Stir in the rice and bring to a boil again. Lower the heat to low, cover, and simmer for about 30 minutes. Stir the vegetables into the fully cooked rice. Sprinkle in the ginger and fluff the mixture. Remove from the heat and keep covered for 15 minutes, allowing the ginger flavor and its benefits to permeate the rice.

YIELD: 4 servings

❓ **How it works:** The carbohydrates in rice help settle the stomach. Carrots, broccoli, and peppers are filled with vitamin B6, and ginger is a vetted antinausea agent.

Note: Eating garlic is safe during pregnancy. However, if the smell or taste of garlic makes you queasy, leave it out.

Nausea-Quelling Ginger Tea

2 cups (475 ml) water
1 teaspoon (3 g) grated fresh ginger, or ½ teaspoon dried
Honey or agave nectar

PREPARATION AND USE:
Bring the water to a boil in a small saucepan. Lower the heat to low. Add
the ginger. Simmer for 5 minutes. Cover and steep for 15 minutes. Strain.
Add sweetener, as desired. Sip over the course of the day.

YIELD: 2 servings

❓ How it works: A half-dozen studies support the use of ginger for nausea
and vomiting during pregnancy. One study in pregnant women found that
ginger was nearly as effective as the antinausea drug metoclopramide (Reglan)
and another found it was as effective as dimenhydrinate (Dramamine). Study
doses have not exceeded 1 gram a day (usually divided into four doses) of
encapsulated ginger nor have they continued past the first trimester.

Homemade Lemon Ginger Ale

Ginger ale is a longstanding stomach settler. But it needs to be made with real ginger. Start with the Nausea-Quelling Ginger Tea recipe (page 80), and add the following ingredients. Experiment with how much honey and lemon you like.

2 cups Nausea-Quelling Ginger Tea
   (page 80, but use twice the amount of ginger)
1 cup (235 ml) carbonated water (Sparkling mineral water works well.)
2 to 3 teaspoons (10 to 15 ml) fresh lemon juice
2 to 3 tablespoons (40 to 60 g) honey

PREPARATION AND USE:
Make the ginger tea as directed. Stir in the carbonated water, lemon, and honey. Sip.

YIELD: 3 servings

How it works: As noted previously, ginger reduces nausea and vomiting during pregnancy. The honey and fresh lemon juice provide potassium, which vomiting can deplete. Lemon contains antioxidant, immune-boosting flavonoids and vitamin C. Honey also provides sugars.

Manipulate Aromas

Strong odors often trigger nausea and vomiting. During my second pregnancy, I couldn't shop at mainstream supermarkets, which seemed suddenly to reek of popcorn, chewing gum, and synthetic fragrances. As an antidote, carry this instant scent-reliever in your bag. ~ LBW

4 drops spearmint essential oil

PREPARATION AND USE:

Place a cotton ball in a 1-ounce (28 ml) bottle. Drop in the spearmint essential oil. Cap. Open and inhale the scent as needed. If you have an aromatherapy diffuser, you can use it to deliver scents into the air.

YIELD: Multiple applications

❓ **How it works:** Some plant aromas have actually been studied as treatments for nausea and vomiting. For instance, essential oils of peppermint, spearmint, ginger, and cardamom reduce postoperative nausea. Although nurse midwives commonly recommend aromatherapy to pregnant women, studies have not yet evaluated effectiveness. The most important thing is that the essential oil smells good to you.

Note: Pregnant women can apply essential oils during pregnancy, but should cut the concentration in half. If a recipe calls for 10 drops of essential oil blended into a carrier oil, use 5 drops instead. Kathi Keville and Mindy Green, authors of *Aromatherapy: A Complete Guide to the Healing Art*, recommend that pregnant women stick to essential oils derived from flowers. Examples include rose, ylang-ylang, German and Roman chamomile, and citrus (bergamot, mandarin, orange, lemon, lime, and neroli). Spearmint and sandalwood are also okay.

Scented, Soothing Spearmint and Chamomile Tea

Chamomile and spearmint are easy to grow. But you can also find them in bulk in natural food stores and in tea bag form.

2 cups (475 ml) water
2 teaspoons (1 g) dried spearmint leaves
2 teaspoons (1 g) dried chamomile flowers

PREPARATION AND USE:

Boil the water. Add the spearmint and chamomile. Steep, covered, for 15 minutes. Strain and sip.

YIELD: 2 servings

❓ **How it works:** Spearmint's soothing aroma and chamomile's antispasmodic qualities also may help quell rising nausea.

Note: Alternatively, boil 2 cups (475 ml) of water and dunk in one spearmint tea bag and one chamomile tea bag.

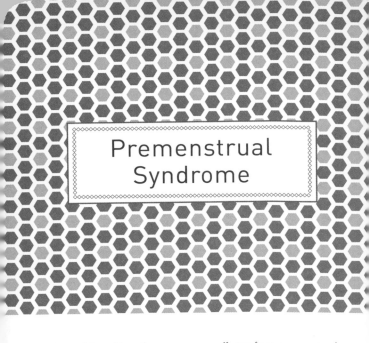

Premenstrual Syndrome

A comic rendition of how fierce a woman suffering from premenstrual syndrome (PMS) can be was well portrayed in the 1990s sitcom *Mad About You*, when the protagonist's younger sister was allowed to go home alone in New York City—armed with PMS and a stun gun.

The moods that sometimes result from PMS can indeed be formidable. Yet, during their reproductive years, some 80 percent of young women have to cope with premenstrual syndrome (PMS). In up to 8 percent, PMS is incapacitating. Happily, for most women, symptoms are mild.

PMS describes a cluster of symptoms that gang up on a woman in the days before her periods only to ebb at the onset of menstrual flow. They include fluid retention, abdominal bloating, headaches, breast tenderness, low back pain, constipation or diarrhea, fatigue, insomnia, sugar cravings, forgetfulness, irritability, decreased self-esteem, social withdrawal, anxiety, and mild depression.

PMS symptoms can cluster into subgroups, depending upon whether the predominant complaint is fluid retention, carbohydrate cravings, anxiety, or depression. A severe form of PMS called premenstrual dysphoric disorder (PMDD) causes marked psychological symptoms: irritability, mood swings, depressed mood, and nervous tension.

The cause of PMS remains a medical mystery. Clearly, monthly oscillations in reproductive hormones have something to do with it. Risk factors include psychological stress, being overweight, and smoking. Doctors sometimes prescribe hormonal contraceptives to smooth out the normal fluctuations in estrogen and progesterone and, occasionally, diuretics to reduce fluid retention and breast tenderness. Antidepressants, either given continuously or only during the last two weeks of the monthly cycle, are helpful for PMDD and when psychological symptoms predominate the PMS picture.

Pre-Attack Snack Mix

¼ cup (36 g) raw almonds

¼ cup (25 g) raw walnut halves

¼ cup (35 g) raisins

¼ cup (21 g) banana chips

¼ cup (21 g) dried apple slices or

(32.5 g) apricots

¼ cup (44 g) carob chips

PREPARATION AND USE:

Preheat the oven to 350°F (180°C, or gas mark 4). Mix the nuts and spread on a baking sheet. Toast for about 10 minutes, stirring after 5 minutes. Remove from the oven, let cool, and pour into a bowl. Toss in the dried fruit and carob chips. Store in an airtight container.

YIELD: 6 servings

❓ **How it works:** Low blood sugar (hypoglycemia) is thought to account for at least some PMS symptoms. Keeping your blood sugar steady with healthy snacks can also help you resist sugar cravings.

PMS Super Salad

1 cup (47 g) torn romaine lettuce

1 cup (28 g) torn red leaf lettuce

½ cup (50 g) torn escarole

½ cup (10 g) torn arugula

⅓ red onion, sliced thinly

½ red bell pepper, seeded and sliced thinly

4 cherry tomatoes

2 tablespoons (30 ml) olive oil

1½ teaspoons (8 ml) balsamic vinegar

1 tablespoon (15 ml) fresh lemon juice

Pinch of freshly ground black pepper

PREPARATION AND USE:

Toss together the leafy greens. Add the onion, bell pepper, and tomatoes. In a separate small bowl, beat together the oil, vinegar, and lemon juice to make a vinaigrette. Add a pinch of black pepper. Drizzle over the greens and toss. Serve.

YIELD: 2 large or 4 small servings

❓ How it works: Some health experts believe that high-fiber, low fat diets may reduce PMS symptoms. In theory, such diets improve elimination of estrogen. The fats to avoid are hydrogenated (trans) fats (in many processed foods) and fat subjected to high heat (present in chips and other fried foods). Healthy fats include monounsaturated fats (e.g., olive oil) and polyunsaturated fats (flaxseed oil, fish oil, evening primrose oil, borage seed oil, and black currant seed oil), which benefit you by reducing inflammation.

Juice It Away

1 cup (235 ml) low-sodium tomato or V8 juice

1 cup (30 g) torn baby spinach, rinsed and drained

1 cup (67 g) torn kale

Salt-free herbal seasoning, such as

½ teaspoon (0.5 g) herbes de Provence

Freshly ground black pepper

PREPARATION AND USE:

Pour the tomato juice into a blender. Gradually add the spinach and kale, mincing it a little at a time so the leaves don't clog the blades. Once minced, blend at high speed to fully pulverize the greens into a liquid. Add more tomato juice if the mixture is too thick. Pour in a tall glass and season to taste with salt-free seasoning and black pepper.

YIELD: 2 servings (about 2 cups [475 ml])

❓ **How it works:** In addition to providing fiber, dark green leafy vegetables contain calcium and magnesium. Low levels of these two minerals are one of the postulated theories about the cause of PMS.

Friendly Fat Salmon-Flax-Avocado Melt

1 can salmon, (4.5 ounces, or 127.5 g) drained

¼ cup (30 g) diced celery

1 tablespoon (10 g) minced red onion

1 teaspoon (4 g) coarsely ground flaxseeds

1 tablespoon (15 g) low-fat plain yogurt

1 teaspoon (5 ml) wine vinegar

Freshly ground black pepper

2 slices whole wheat bread

½ avocado, peeled, pitted, and sliced

PREPARATION AND USE:

In a bowl, mix together the salmon, celery, onion, flaxseeds, yogurt, and vinegar. Top each slice of bread with half of the salmon mixture. Spray a skillet lightly with canola oil cooking spray. Cook the open-faced sandwiches over low heat for about 5 minutes until the bread is toasty. Top each sandwich with the avocado slices.

YIELD: 2 servings

❓ **How it works:** Some studies have shown that the omega-3 fatty acids found in fish oils, avocado, nuts, flaxseeds, and olive oil can help reduce bloating and discomfort associated with PMS. One recent study showed that women who ate 25 grams of flaxseeds every day had reduced premenstrual breast pain. A possible explanation is that flaxseeds contain lignans, which act as phytoestrogens (natural estrogen-like substances).

B-Rich Burritos

3 cups (516 g) cooked pinto beans

1 cup (260 g) salsa

3 tablespoons (30 g) chopped onion

1 cup (195 g) cooked brown rice

1 ripe avocado, pitted, peeled, and sliced

8 tortillas, preferably whole wheat

PREPARATION AND USE:

Mix together the beans, salsa, onion, and rice. Fill each tortilla with about 3 tablespoons (185 g) of the mixture. Top with avocado.

YIELD: 8 servings

? How it works: Several of the B vitamins, including B6, are needed to make brain chemicals, some of which influence mood and may have to do with PMS. A recent study found that women who consume more B vitamins from food sources had a lower risk of PMS. Beans, lentils, whole grains, avocados, and bananas are good sources.

Nutty Rice Regulator

This delicious and textured recipe delivers the magnesium and B vitamins that can help block PMS.

1½ cups (292 g) uncooked brown rice

1 cup (100 g) crushed almonds

1 cup (240 g) canned chickpeas, drained and rinsed

2½ cups (570 ml) water

1 tablespoon (15 ml) olive oil

1 teaspoon (1 g) salt-free herbal seasoning

2 garlic cloves, crushed

PREPARATION AND USE:

Preheat the oven to 375°F (190°C, or gas mark 5). Stir together the rice, almonds, and chickpeas, and pour into a medium-size glass baking dish. In a saucepan, bring the water, olive oil, and seasoning to a boil. Pour the boiling water over the rice mixture and stir. Stir in the crushed garlic. Cover the dish tightly with aluminum foil. Bake for 1 hour on the oven's middle rack.

YIELD: 6 to 8 servings

❓ **How it works:** Brown rice and almonds are among the foods highest in magnesium content, supplying a hearty 100 milligrams per serving. Supplemental magnesium has been shown to help with mood swings and fluid retention during PMS. Chickpeas are high in B vitamins, which also help reduce PMS.

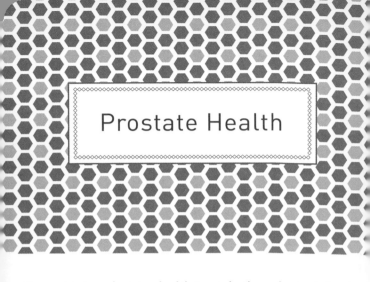

Prostate Health

The prostate is a walnut-size gland that encircles the urethra just below the bladder. Glandular tissue contributes fluid to the semen; muscles within the prostate help expel semen during ejaculation.

Disorders of the prostate are relatively common. More than 30 million men suffer from prostate conditions, such as prostatitis, benign prostatic hyperplasia, and prostate cancer. The first is more common in younger men; the last two become more common with age.

Prostatitis (prostate inflammation) affects about half of men sometime during their lifetime. Bacteria can infect the prostate gland. The prostate is also susceptible to acute and chronic noninfectious inflammation, though the underlying cause is poorly understood.

The symptoms of acute bacterial prostatitis include frequent and painful urination, pain in the low back or behind the testicles, painful ejaculation, aching muscles, fever, chills, and fatigue. Chronic bacterial infection can cause mild symptoms or none at all. Noninfectious prostatitis mainly causes pelvic pain, as well as pain with ejaculation and urination.

Bacterial prostatitis is treated with antibiotics. Treatment of noninfectious prostatitis is more challenging. Pain relievers, a class of medication called beta-blockers, and physical therapy may help.

Benign prostatic hyperplasia, also called benign prostatic hypertrophy (BPH), affects mostly older men. About half of fifty- to sixty-year-old men develop BPH. Between ages eighty and ninety that proportion rises to,nearly 90 percent. This noncancerous enlargement of the prostate encroaches on the urethra, decreasing the ability of urine to easily flow from the bladder. Symptoms include increased frequency and urgency of urination, nighttime urination, a weak urine stream, an inability to fully empty the bladder, and difficulty stopping and starting urination.

The underlying cause is an age-related rise in prostate levels of dihydrotestosterone (DHT) as well as estrogen, which stimulate cells to multiply.

Prescription medications can reduce prostate size and improve urine flow. Severe cases may require surgery.

Super Tomatillo-Pumpkin Seed Salad Dressing

1 can (13 ounces, or 368 g) tomatillos, drained

½ white onion, chopped

¼ cup (4 g) fresh cilantro leaves, chopped

½ cup (32 g) roasted pumpkin seeds

1 jalapeño pepper, seeded and chopped

1 garlic clove

1 tablespoon (15 ml) fresh lime juice

Water

Salt

PREPARATION AND USE:

Purée the first seven ingredients in a blender until coarse. Pour in a bowl and add just enough water to give it a saucelike consistency. Add salt to taste. Drizzle over broiled chicken or fish.

YIELD: 4 servings

❓ **How it works:** Pumpkin seeds contain healthy oil, fiber, carotenes (which are antioxidant and promote immune function), vitamin E, and zinc. Pumpkin seed oil extracts, with or without saw palmetto, can reduce BPH symptoms. Zinc seems to inhibit proliferation of prostate cancer cells. Low zinc can occur in men with BPH and prostate cancer. Zinc is also needed for sperm production.

Salubrious Stir-Fried Veggies and Tofu

1 cup (248 g) firm tofu, cubed
1½ teaspoons (8 ml) soy sauce
3 tablespoons (45 ml) olive oil, divided
3 cups (400 g) combination of any of the
following: chopped red bell pepper,
asparagus, onion, broccoli, and mushrooms
3 garlic cloves, minced
1½ teaspoons (4 g) grated fresh ginger
Freshly ground black pepper

PREPARATION AND USE:

In a bowl, toss together tofu, soy sauce, and 1 tablespoon (15 ml) of the olive oil. Heat a skillet over medium-high and sauté the coated tofu about 3 minutes until it begins to brown. Transfer the tofu to a bowl and set aside. Into the hot skillet place the remaining olive oil, veggies, garlic, and ginger. Sauté the mix for about 6 minutes. Add the tofu and combine it with the vegetables. Add black pepper to taste. Enjoy the veggies in a bowl or over brown rice.

YIELD: 3 to 4 servings

❓ **How it works:** Traditional Asian diets are associated with a reduced likelihood of BPH and prostate cancer. These diets include regular consumption of vegetables, soy, and green tea, all of which contain substances that restrain prostate growth. On the other hand, diets high in fats, carbohydrates, and red meat seem to increase the risk.

Powerful Pomegranate Smoothie

2 cups (400 g) plain nonfat Greek yogurt

8 ounces (235 ml) pure pomegranate juice

1 banana, peeled, cut into chunks, and frozen

½ cup (128 g) sliced strawberries, frozen

PREPARATION AND USE:

Pour the yogurt and juice into a blender. Add the fruit and blend until smooth. Enjoy!

YIELD: 2 servings

❓ **How it works:** Pomegranate juice inhibits the development of prostate cancer and the progression of already existent prostate cancer. Compounds in pomegranate cause prostate cancer cells to die and decrease the migration of these cells. A study in men with prostate cancer resulted in none of the patients progressing to advanced stages while drinking 8 ounces (235 ml) of pomegranate juice a day. Pomegranate also slowed the rise in blood levels of PSA.

Broiled Tomatoes with Beneficial Garlic

3 large round tomatoes (not Roma or plum)

3 large garlic cloves

2 teaspoons (2 g) crushed dried thyme leaves

Freshly ground black pepper

¼ cup (60 ml) olive oil

1 tablespoon (10 g) crushed garlic

Warm, crusty loaf of whole-grain bread

PREPARATION AND USE:

Preheat the oven to broil. Cut each tomato in half across its equator. Place the tomato halves face up on a baking sheet. Slice the garlic cloves lengthwise to make six pieces and insert a piece into each of the tomatoes. Sprinkle each tomato half with thyme and pepper. Drizzle with oil. Broil for about 10 minutes. After broiling, dot the tomatoes with the crushed garlic (broiling tends to deactivate benefits of the inserted garlic). Serve with warm, crusty bread.

YIELD: 6 servings

❓ **How it works:** Studies in the early part of the twenty-first century linked high intake of tomato products (and the lycopene they contain) with a lower risk of prostate cancer. A few years later, however, the correlation failed to hold up. Nevertheless, tomatoes and other plant foods contain a host of nutrients beneficial to health. One study found that garlic extracts improve urine flow in men with BPH and prostate cancer. Garlic also enhances immune function and has anti-prostate-cancer activity.

Antioxidant Orange Cranberry Muffins

2 cups (180 g) oat flour

2 teaspoons (9 g) baking powder

1 cup (110 g) chopped pecans or (120 g) walnuts

2 teaspoons (5 g) flaxseed meal

½ cup (120 ml) canola oil

1 cup (235 ml) fresh orange juice

3 tablespoons (60 g) honey or agave nectar

1 cup (120 g) coarsely chopped dried cranberries

PREPARATION AND USE:

Preheat the oven to 350°F (180°C, or gas mark 4). Grease a twelve-compartment muffin tin or line it with paper liners. In a large bowl, mix the oat flour, baking powder, pecans, and flaxseed meal. Pour the oil, orange juice, and honey into the flour mixture and stir until just moistened. Fold in the cranberries. Do not overmix. Spoon the batter into the prepared muffin tin. Bake for about 25 minutes, or until a toothpick inserted into the center of a muffin comes out clean. Transfer the muffin tin to a cooling rack and cool for 5 minutes.

YIELD: 10 to 12 muffins

❓ **How it works:** Cranberry contains potent antioxidant and anti-inflammatory substances, which helps prevent bacterial urinary tract infections in women. One study found that dried, powdered cranberries (500 milligrams three times a day for six months) ameliorated symptoms in men with chronic nonbacterial prostatitis. A test-tube study found that cranberry extract inhibited growth of human prostate cancer cells.

The Big Q Baked Onion

The big Q—quercetin—is a prostate protector. You'll find quercetin in onions, citrus fruits, apples, parsley, sage, tea, red wine, and olive oil.

2 Vidalia onions

Olive oil

¼ cup (7 g) whole fresh rosemary leaves

Freshly ground black pepper

PREPARATION AND USE:

Preheat the oven to 350°F (180°C, or gas mark 4). Place two squares of aluminum foil, each large enough to wrap an onion, on a baking sheet. Leave the skins on the Vidalias and cut out the stems, making an indentation about an inch (2.5 cm) deep and wide on each onion. Place each onion on a foil square. Baste each onion indentation with olive oil. Sprinkle pepper into the indentation and fill it with whole rosemary leaves. Enclose each onion in the foil and pinch the top together. Bake for about 1 hour. The onions should be tender and easy to pierce with a fork. Remove them from the aluminum foil and peel before serving.

YIELD: 2 to 4 servings

❓ How it works: Quercetin— an antioxidant found in many plants— and other flavonoids seem to protect against several cancers, including prostate cancer. In one study, supplemental quercetin (500 milligrams twice daily for one month) reduced symptoms of chronic nonbacterial prostatitis. In onions, the quercetin is concentrated in the skin, so keep the skin intact while baking and remove afterward. In addition to onions, quercetin comes in flavonoid-rich fruits, such as grapes, dark cherries, blackberries, bilberries, and blueberries.

Muscle-Toning Kegel Exercises

These exercises improve the tone of the pelvic floor muscles and may reduce urinary symptoms of prostatitis and improve urinary continence after surgical removal of the prostate.

You

A rug or comfortable pad

PREPARATION AND USE:

First, locate the pelvic floor muscles, which are below the bladder; the easiest time to identify them is during urination. (You use the same muscles to stop yourself from passing gas.) Partway through urination, purposely contract those muscles to stop the flow of urine without holding your breath or tensing the other muscles in your abdomen, legs, or buttocks. When you successfully interrupt the flow, you have located the correct muscles. Also, the contraction causes your testicles and base of your penis to rise. From now on, perform Kegels when you're not urinating. Doing it while urinating may weaken, rather than strengthen, pelvic floor muscles.

Next: With an empty bladder, lie flat on your back on the rug or pad. Counting to five, slowly contract the pelvic floor muscles you have located above.Counting to five again, slowly relax the pelvic floor muscles. Repeat this pair of movements ten times for one full set. Practice three full sets daily. Gradually, within a month, work up to counting to ten as you contract and relax the muscles. Work up to five sets daily. As your muscles become stronger, do the exercise in a standing position. This will increase your muscle control.

YIELD: Multiple sessions

❓ How it works: In men, urinary incontinence can be caused by a weak urinary sphincter that may result from surgery for prostate cancer, an overactive bladder, or a bladder that doesn't contract. By toning the pelvic floor muscles beneath the bladder, Kegel exercises can help you improve—or in some cases completely regain—bladder control. They help control urination and curb dribbling and incontinence.

Note: Focus only on tensing the pelvic floor muscles. Try to keep your other muscles—abdomen, legs, and buttocks—relaxed during Kegels. If a month has passed and the symptoms haven't improved, it may be a sign that you're not exercising the right muscles. Ask your doctor for help locating them.

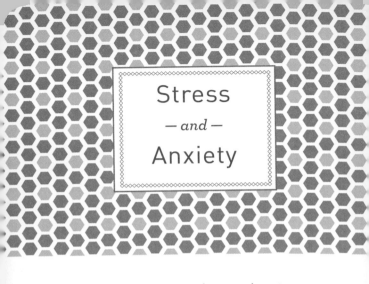

Stress
—and—
Anxiety

Perhaps you've had the dream. You're about to make an important presentation. Everything seems perfect—until you look down and realize you're not wearing any pants.

Sometimes anxiety bubbles up in our sleep. Or it manifests as muscle tension—the clenched jaw, furrowed brow, and tight shoulders. Anxiety can cause headaches, stomach upset, worried thoughts, insomnia, and other symptoms. Psychological stress is the most common cause of transient and low-level anxiety.

Unfortunately, stress is all too common in America. Surveys show that about one-third of people feel routinely overwhelmed by stress. Worse, many stressed people use unhealthy means to manage it. Experts in the field have called stress overload a public health crisis.

Paradoxically, the stress response damages health but is essential to survival. It's supremely designed to help us survive physical stressors. Confrontation with a saber-toothed tiger (or other threat) inspires alarm. Ancient brain areas activate the sympathetic nervous system (fight or-flight response) and two adrenal hormones: epinephrine (adrenaline) and cortisol (related to the drug cortisone).

The end result is increased blood sugar, heart rate, breathing rate, and blood pressure. Dilation of arteries to the brain, heart, and muscles ensures the delivery of oxygen and glucose-rich blood. Blood vessels to other organs constrict and activity of those organs (e.g., the intestinal tract) declines. Basically, a crisis is not the time to digest lunch.

The biological situation is perfect—if you are fighting or fleeing a predator. It's not so good if you're caught in a traffic jam and late for an important date. All that palpitating will only hurt your health.

Chronic stress overload raises the risk for a number of conditions that commonly plague Americans. They include high blood pressure, atherosclerosis, heart disease, diabetes, immune system dysfunction, increased sensitivity to pain, and fatigue. Chronic stress contributes to stomach ulcers, indigestion, and irritable bowel syndrome. It throws a wet blanket over sexual desire and can interfere with menstrual cycles. It makes us crave high-calorie food and store fat in our abdomens. It disrupts sleep, impairs learning and memory, and renders us irritable and moody. Over the long haul, stress accelerates aging.

RECIPES TO PREVENT AND MANAGE STRESS AND ANXIETY

De-Stress Journal

You

A journal

A pen

PREPARATION AND USE:

Write about one incident in your recent past that made you feel stressed. Record your thoughts, emotions, and bodily sensations: Did you feel angry and blame others? Helpless? Resigned to the situation? Did you feel tightness, pain, or tension in your body? If so, where? Record the steps you took to address the stress: Did you light a cigarette? Have a drink? Go outside? Call a friend? Slam doors? Next, record daily stressful incidents and your reactions for a week. At the end of the week, review the journal and identify your patterns of reaction. Zero in on one or two reactions that you feel are especially harmful to your mental or physical health and that you want to change.

YIELD: Daily session

❓ **How it works:** The purpose of this exercise is to recognize how you respond to stress. The way we react to daily hassles becomes ingrained and automatic. The goal isn't to avoid stress altogether (which would be impossible and not even truly desirable), but to respond in ways that serve you. Awareness is the first step toward changing unhealthy habits and maximizing the skills that are working for you.

Visualize Confidence

You

A quiet place

PREPARATION AND USE:

In a quiet place, visualize a forthcoming situation that you think will cause you stress: a presentation, a discussion with an estranged loved one, or an exam. Visualize the optimal way you can address this challenge. Imagine yourself feeling calm and focused and others responding positively to you. Prepare for the event, and then let it go (do not let your mind return to it). Enter the situation with confidence and address it as you have visualized. You will be surprised at the outcome. And, keep in mind that it's normal to feel performance anxiety.

YIELD: 1 session

❓ How it works: By imagining the strongest outcome for a challenging situation, you can prepare for and enter it with confidence and calm. Even if the results aren't exactly what you've envisioned, they will likely be more successful than if you'd anticipated conflict and defeat. Addressing a situation with a positive outlook usually brings positive results.

LIFESTYLE TIP

Avoid turning to alcohol, sedatives, tobacco, and junk food for stress relief. They might bring you a fleeting release. However, all of these substances actually aggravate stress. Substitute such habits with healthier alternatives, such as those suggested in the remedies in this chapter.

Super Senses Mindfulness

You

An apple or other piece of fruit

PREPARATION AND USE:

Sit quietly. Hold the apple, polish it, smell it, feel its contours, look carefully at its color, its blemishes, and its beauty. Anticipate eating it. Bite into the apple. Slowly, deliberately chew it, savoring the burst of flavor. Don't swallow it immediately, but try to identify the different kinds of tastes and scents you are experiencing. What thoughts are going through your mind? Does eating this apple remind you of pleasant memories?

YIELD: 1 session

❓ **How it works:** This mindfulness exercise stimulates the senses, guiding you to more deeply appreciate the world right in front of you and the simple things that make it up.

Nerve-Calming Aroma Relief

Choosing to surround yourself with a scent will link you with situations in which you've felt peaceful. Essential oil of your favorite aroma (choose from lavender, chamomile, rose, jasmine, bergamot, or neroli)

PREPARATION AND USE:

Fill a bathtub with warm water. Drop in 10 to 12 drops of your choice of essential oil. Disperse the oil with your hand. Luxuriate.

YIELD: 1 application

❓ How it works: Aromas are relayed to those ancient brain areas that trigger the stress response. Emerging research shows that some plant essential oils reduce objective and subjective measurements of stress and anxiety. Examples include German and Roman chamomile, lavender, rose, and jasmine.

Note: Other options for aroma use: Diffuse it or add it to lotion, using 10 to 12 drops per ounce (28 ml).

Destressing Aroma Inhaler

Your favorite essential oil

PREPARATION AND USE:
Drop a few drops of your favorite oil on a cotton ball. Place the ball in a clean jar and cap it. Open the jar and inhale the aroma when you are in any stressful situation.

YIELD: Multiple applications

❓ **How it works:** Some plant essential oils help reduce stress and feelings of anxiety. Carry this inhaler with you for immediate stress relief.

LIFESTYLE TIP

Reach out. A famous University of California, Los Angeles study suggested that while men may be programmed for fight or flight, women are more likely to follow a "tend-and-befriend" pattern when stressed. Hugging releases oxytocin, a bonding hormone that counteracts stress. Men have it, too!

Sereni-Tea

1 cup (26 g) dried lemon balm leaves

¼ cup (6 g) dried German chamomile flowers

2 tablespoons (3 g) dried lavender flowers

2 tablespoons (3 g) dried rosebuds or petals

¼ cup (6 g) dried passionflower

2 cups (475 ml) water

Stevia or honey (optional)

PREPARATION AND USE:

Mix the dried herbs and place them in a clean jar. Boil the water in a pot. Remove from the heat. Add 2 tablespoons (3 g) of the mixture and cover. Steep 15 minutes. Strain and serve. Add stevia or honey if you want it sweeter. Sip and relax.

YIELD: 2 small servings

How it works: All of these herbs calm the nervous system. Most of the herbs have been studied in the laboratory. One study found a special extract of German chamomile helped people with generalized anxiety disorder.

Note: All measurements are for dried plants. If you use fresh, double the amounts. If you don't have access to bulk herbs, buy chamomile tea bags or a tea blend of some of these herbs. Other calming herbs include hops, skullcap, and valerian. All act as gentle sedatives. Reserve stronger herbs, such as hops and valerian, until closer to bedtime.

Ulcers

As commonplace as they seem, stomach ulcers have caused pain, illness, and even premature death. Take Charles Darwin, who attributed his constant stomach problems to seasickness. Doctors now suspect he was infected with the ulcer-causing bacterium *Helicobacter pylori*. Stomach ulcers, combined with a parasitic infection that damaged his heart, contributed to his ill chronic health and death at age seventy-three.

By definition, an ulcer is an erosion on any bodily surface—the skin or the mucous membranes that line hollow organs. When people use the word, they're usually referring to peptic ulcers, in which case the craterlike sores occur in the stomach or duodenum (first part of the small intestine). However, ulcers can occur anywhere along the gastrointestinal tract, from mouth to anus.

Let's start with the mouth. Canker sores (also called aphthous ulcers) are the most common problem. These small, but painful sores usually heal within seven to ten days. Genetic vulnerability seems to play a role. Triggers include food allergies, stress, smoking, trauma (from braces, dentures, hot foods, or hard toothbrushes), certain medications, toothpastes containing sodium lauryl sulfate, and nutrient deficiencies (vitamin C, vitamin B12, folic acid, and iron).

A different entity altogether, fever blisters (also called cold sores) occur on the lips, are caused by herpes simplex virus, and are very contagious.

A more serious condition is inflammatory bowel disease. This category includes ulcerative colitis and Crohn's disease. In ulcerative colitis, the inflammation and ulcers stay within the colon (large intestine). In Crohn's disease, the entire gastrointestinal tract is vulnerable to ulceration. Both conditions require careful medical management.

Back to gastric (stomach) ulcers. The problem often begins with gastritis, inflammation of the stomach. Causes include alcohol abuse, nonsteroidal anti-inflammatory drugs (aspirin, ibuprofen, naproxen), and infection with the bacterium *Helicobacter pylori*. The condition may lack symptoms or produce upper abdominal pain, nausea, and vomiting. If an ulcer develops, signs of bleeding include black, tarry stools, red blood in the stool, or bloody vomitus.

H. pylori is now considered the main cause of peptic ulcers. The bacterium is present in the majority of people with ulcers. However, only 20 percent of people infected with *H. pylori* develop ulcers. Clearly, other factors contribute.

Cabbage Juice Relief

Cabbage juice is a long-standing folk medicine against peptic ulcers. During the early 1950s, Garnett Cheney, MD, conducted research on "vitamin U," an antiulcer factor in raw cabbage juice.

½ head white cabbage, washed and chopped coarsely (no hearts)

About 2 cups (475 ml) water

PREPARATION AND USE:

Fill a blender with the cabbage. Add water to the two-thirds mark. Blend on high speed until fully blended, about a minute. Strain or press the mixture. (A medium-size French press works well to strain out the juice.) Drink ½ cup (120 ml) up to three times a day. Store the unused portion in the refrigerator. Discard after twenty-four hours.

YIELD: 12 ounces (355 ml) cabbage juice

❓ **How it works:** In the 1950s, Cheney and colleagues conducted a study on San Quentin Prison inmates that demonstrated improved healing of peptic ulcers from concentrated cabbage juice relative to a placebo beverage. Volunteers received 50 milliliters (just under 2 ounces, or ¼ cup) a day for twenty-one days. Later research showed that the fresh juice of white cabbage stimulates the immune system and contains glutamine, an amino acid that may improve the stomach's protective lining.

Breakfast Boost

Studies show that fasting during Ramadan increases stomach acidity and increases the odds of ulcer reactivation. Aside from religious fasting, many people skip breakfast. This simple, healthful breakfast boost has ingredients that inhibit H. pylori *bacteria.*

1 large banana, frozen and sliced

1 cup (255 g) frozen sliced strawberries

1 cup (230 g) vanilla yogurt

3 tablespoons (36 g) psyllium powder

1 to 2 cups (235 to 475 ml) cranberry or cranapple juice

PREPARATION AND USE:

In a blender, blend together the bananas, strawberries, and yogurt. Blend in the psyllium powder. Add the juice to your desired consistency and amount

YIELD: 2 servings

❓ How it works: A bacterium common in fermented dairy products (*Lactobacillus acidophilus*) produces fatty acids that suppress *H. pylori*. In test-tube studies, cranberry extract and honey inhibit *H. pylori*.

Wrap-It-Up Fish

2 long sheets (about 13 x 18-inches [33 x 45.5 cm]) phyllo pastry

1 tablespoon (15 ml) olive oil

½ zucchini, chopped

8 broccoli florets, halved

1 garlic clove, minced

1 salmon fillet (8 ounces, or 225 g), skin removed

1 tablespoon (10 ml) vegetable stock

1 teaspoon (10 g) chopped dill

PREPARATION AND USE:

Preheat the oven to 350°F (180°C, or gas mark 4). Lightly spray a large baking sheet with cooking spray. Spread out one phyllo sheet on the prepared baking sheet. Lightly brush the phyllo sheet with olive oil. Place the second sheet on top of the first and lightly brush with olive oil. Cover the top layer of phyllo with a layer of zucchini and broccoli. Sprinkle with the garlic. Lay the salmon on top. Spoon the vegetable stock over the salmon. Sprinkle the dill on top. Fold up the phyllo pastry, envelope style, to cover the salmon and pinch together the edges. Lightly brush the outside of the packet with olive oil. Bake for 20 minutes.

YIELD: 2 servings

❓ **How it works:** Some polyunsaturated fatty acids, including the kind in fish oil, evening primrose oil, flaxseed oil, and black currant seed oil, are anti-inflammatory and inhibit *H. pylori*. A type of fatty acid prominent in oily fish, such as salmon, may be particularly helpful. In test-tube studies, garlic inhibits *H. pylori*.

Mouth Ulcer Paste

1 teaspoon (5 g) baking soda
Water

PREPARATION AND USE:

In a small, clean dish, mix together the baking soda and as much water as needed to form a paste. With a cotton swab, apply to each sore to your desired thickness. Create a fresh batch and apply three times a day.

YIELD: 1 application

? How it works: The baking soda paste covers the sore to protect it from irritants. The Mayo Clinic recommends this mixture to ease pain and help healing.

Alternate: For a quick rinse, mix 1 cup (235 ml) of warm water, ¼ teaspoon of baking soda, and $^1/8$ teaspoon of salt. Rinse several times a day using a new batch each time. Then rinse with a plain cup (235 ml) of water.

Slippery Elm Mouth Ulcer Relief

1 tablespoon (15 g) Aloe vera gel

1 teaspoon (5 g) powdered slippery elm bark

PREPARATION AND USE:

Put both ingredients in a small, clean jar and blend with a chopstick. Dot on mouth ulcers as needed. Cap the jar when not in use.

YIELD: Multiple applications

❓ How it works: Aloe vera gel decreases inflammation, stimulates the immune system, and enhances wound healing. Preliminary studies show that topical aloe gel decreases the pain of aphthous ulcers and speeds healing. The inner bark of slippery elm (*Ulmus rubra*) contains mucilaginous substances that coat and soothe irritated membranes.

Note: Use either 99 percent aloe gel or fresh aloe gel gently scraped from the inner leaf of an Aloe vera plant (we recommend growing one in an indoor pot). You can find powdered slipper elm bark at natural food stores and herb retailers.

Positively Pleasing Ulcer Potion

6 cups (1.4 L) water

¼ cup (25 g) fresh ginger slices

6 chamomile tea bags

1 tablespoon (3 g) chopped fresh sage

3 cups (700 ml) pure cranberry juice

Honey (optional)

PREPARATION AND USE:

Boil the water in a large pot. Add the ginger, tea bags, and sage; steep for 10 minutes. Strain into a pitcher. Stir in the juice. Add honey, if desired. Drink throughout the day.

YIELD: 8 servings

❓ **How it works:** In test-tube studies, chamomile and sage inhibit H. pylori. Cranberry and honey are inhibitors as well. Animal studies indicate that ginger reduces the concentration of H. pylori and inflammation in the stomach and protects against stress-induced ulcers. Whether these plants are similarly helpful in humans isn't yet known. However, they all have other health benefits and taste great.

Vaginal Yeast Infections

Vaginitis means inflammation of the vagina. A number of things can irritate the vagina: infections with bacteria, fungi, and protozoa; harsh chemicals in personal care products; and even the loss of estrogen after menopause.

Yeast, a type of fungus, normally colonize the vagina though in small numbers relative to health-promoting bacteria such as lactobacilli. An overgrowth of certain types of yeast, such as *Candida albicans*, produces vaginal yeast infections (also called yeast vaginitis or vaginal candidiasis). Usually the labia and clitoris are also inflamed. About 75 percent of women have at least one episode in their lifetime; 5 to 10 percent have recurrent attacks.

The following factors raise the risk of yeast vaginitis:

- Antibiotics kill the "friendly" bacteria that normally defend the vagina.
- Douches and some vaginal "hygiene" sprays can irritate the vagina and disrupt the microbial ecology.
- Cancer chemotherapy, cortisone like medications, and HIV infection suppress the immune system, allowing disease-causing microbes to flourish.
- Diabetes mellitus raises glucose (sugar) levels in bodily fluids, allowing feasting yeast to proliferate.

Symptoms include itching, burning, a thick white discharge, and discomfort during intercourse. Health professionals diagnose the condition with visual inspection and microscopic examination of the discharge. Treatment centers on intravaginal antifungal creams and suppositories. Oral antifungal drugs may be prescribed for more severe cases. Before you try home remedies or over-the-counter antifungal creams, we recommend you get a medical diagnosis. Women correctly self-diagnose yeast vaginitis only about half the time. Other pathogens that don't respond to antifungal drugs—some with potentially serious complications—can cause similar symptoms or may coexist with the yeast overgrowth.

Home management is only appropriate if you're sure you have yeast and your symptoms are mild. If you're pregnant, do not try any home remedies (with the exception of eating yogurt) without consulting your physician.

Healing Honeyed Yogurt

1 cup (235 ml) water

2 tablespoons (40 g) raw (unprocessed) honey

2 tablespoons (30 g) plain, active-culture yogurt

PREPARATION AND USE:

Boil the water in a kettle or saucepan. Allow it to cool so that it's very warm but not scalding. Place the honey in a bowl. Raw honey can be very thick, so add just enough of the warm water (no more than 1 to 2 teaspoons [5 to 10 ml]) so that you can blend the honey with the yogurt. Add the yogurt and blend thoroughly with a clean spoon. Transfer the mixture to a clean jar. With clean fingers, apply about 1 teaspoon (11.5 g) to the vagina and vulva. (Don't double-dip. If you have a clean vaginal applicator, you can spoon the mixture into it and apply it that way.) Repeat two times a day for seven days. We recommend you wear a panty liner. Store the jar in the refrigerator between applications. Toss after one week.

YIELD: Twelve 1-teaspoon (11.5 g) applications

❓ How it works: Raw honey has antifungal activity. Yogurt contains Lactobacilli, which is the type of bacteria normally found in the vagina. These friendly bacteria promote healthy immune system function and lower pH (more acidic environments are hostile to fungi). In a study published in 2012 in the *Archives of Obstetrics and Gynecology*, researchers created a blend of distilled water, local honey, and yogurt and then assigned pregnant women with yeast vaginitis to use the honey-yogurt blend or topical antifungal cream. Both were effective, but the honey-yogurt blend more so.

Note: Raw honey hasn't been processed or heated, thus retaining all active ingredients.

Intravaginal Yogurt

Plain, active-culture yogurt

PREPARATION AND USE:

Apply to the vagina and vulva two or three times a day.

YIELD: Multiple applications

? **How it works:** Yogurt contains *lactobacilli*, which protect against yeast vaginitis. Despite a long folk tradition, clinical trials have not evaluated intravaginal yogurt used alone for women with recurrent yeast infections. Such use may have more potential value as a preventive rather than a treatment for an active yeast infection. *Lactobacilli* do, however, interfere with the ability of disease-causing bacteria to colonize the vagina.

Fact or Myth?

YEAST VAGINITIS IS A SEXUALLY TRANSMITTED INFECTION.

Not necessarily. Men can pick it up from their female partners, though they less often develop symptoms. However, women who have never had sexual intercourse can develop yeast vaginitis. Yeast, which already exist in the vagina, simply grow out of control.

Garlic Suppository

1 garlic clove, peeled

PREPARATION AND USE:

Wrap the clove in a single layer of sterile gauze and twist, to create a "tail" that's 1 to 2 inches (2.5 to 5 cm) long. (If you have no irritation after the first application, you can gently nick the clove next time.) Insert the gauze-covered clove into the vagina, leaving a small piece of the tail-end of the gauze at the vaginal entrance. (Adding a bit of K-Y Jelly or other lubricant to the end can ease the insertion). Remove after 1 hour. Repeat three times a day.

YIELD: 1 application

❓ **How it works:** Garlic is antimicrobial, with activity against fungi. However, no clinical trials have evaluated this folk remedy.

❗ **Warning:** Prolonged use of topical garlic can irritate skin and mucous membranes. Some people are allergic. Discontinue use if irritation occurs.

Antiyeast Bath

1 cup (235 ml) apple cider vinegar

PREPARATION AND USE:

As you run a warm bath, pour in the apple cider vinegar and disperse it with your hand. Luxuriate for at least 20 minutes as the vinegar works to inhibit yeast growth.

YIELD: 1 application

❓ **How it works:** Vinegar can help arrest the growth of Candida albicans, a common cause of yeast infections. All three essential oil alternatives are antifungal.

Recipe Variation: Add essential oils to your bath, along with the vinegar: tea tree oil, eucalyptus, or, lavender.

Antifungal Wash

2 cups (475 ml) water
1 tablespoon (6 g) green tea
1 tablespoon (3 g) dried rosemary or (2 g) sage
1 tablespoon (15 ml) apple cider vinegar
1 drop tea tree essential oil

PREPARATION AND USE:

Boil the water. Add the tea and rosemary. Cover and steep 15 to 20 minutes. Strain into a jar. Add the vinegar and oil and shake well to disperse the oil. Moisten a tampon with the mixture and insert into the vagina. After 15 minutes, remove the tampon. Wear a panty liner.

❓ How it works: Some natural medicine practitioners use diluted tea tree oil to manage vaginitis. Tea tree essential oil is antimicrobial against a number of organisms, including *Candida albicans*. Ensure that it is diluted as local irritation and allergic reactions are possible. Tea tree essential oil is very strong and should only be applied externally; it can be toxic if ingested. Tea (*Camellia sinensis*), rosemary, and sage are also active against Candida yeast. Vinegar contains acetic acid, which discourages yeast overgrowth.

⚠ Warning: Do not douche or insert tampons while pregnant.

Note: This formula has not been tested in any clinical trial. Alternatively, you can very gently douche with this mixture. Although it's okay to do so if you have a yeast infection, do not continue douching on a regular basis. Doing so can disrupt the normal ecology of vaginal microbes. Be sure to wear a panty liner.

Quickie Kimchi

1 head savoy cabbage

1 cup (110 g) grated carrot

¼ cup (60 g) sea salt

½ teaspoon minced fresh garlic

4 scallions, chopped

1 teaspoon (5 ml) Asian fish sauce

1 tablespoon (13 g) sugar

½ teaspoon ground ginger

2 teaspoons (5.2 g) chili powder, or to taste

PREPARATION AND USE:

Trim the bottom of the cabbage, slice it lengthwise, and cut each half into chunks. Mix together the cabbage chunks and carrot in a large glass bowl. Toss with the salt to coat the vegetable mixture. Cover the bowl securely with plastic wrap and allow to sit at room temperature for 5 to 6 hours. Transfer the mixture from the bowl to a colander, rinse off the salt, and then drain the vegetable mixture, thoroughly, pressing out all the liquid. Return the mixture to the rinsed bowl and stir in all the remaining ingredients, except the chili powder. When all the ingredients are combined, add the chili powder and stir well to coat. You can knead it in by hand, but wear plastic gloves to protect your fingers from the heat. Transfer the mixture to a clean 24-ounce (710 ml) glass jar. Cap the lid tightly. Set the jar in a cool, dry place for four days. Refrigerate, then serve. Refrigerated, the mixture keeps for about four weeks.

? **How it works:** Fermented foods contain probiotics. The intestines are the source of fungi that infect the vagina (and also of the bacteria that cause bladder infections and a non-sexually transmitted vaginal infection called bacterial vaginosis). Disruption in the microbial ecology of the gut (due to antibiotics and other causes) can promote fungal overgrowth in the vagina. Although oral probiotics are unlikely to treat an active yeast infection, regular consumption may help prevent them.

Yogurt and Berries Breakfast Treat

1 cup (230 g) plain nonfat, active-culture yogurt (We like Greek yogurt,
   which has a satisfying thickness even when low in fat.)
¼ cup (36 g) fresh berries (or other favorite fruit)

PREPARATION AND USE:

Scoop the yogurt into a bowl. Top with the berries. Spoon into your mouth
and enjoy.

YIELD: 1 serving

❓ **How it works:** Yogurt contains probiotics, live microorganisms
(mainly bacteria), that promote human health. Regularly eating yogurt
seems to help prevent yeast infections. Active-culture yogurt contains
bacteria normally found in the intestinal tract and vagina. These organisms
promote healthy immune function.

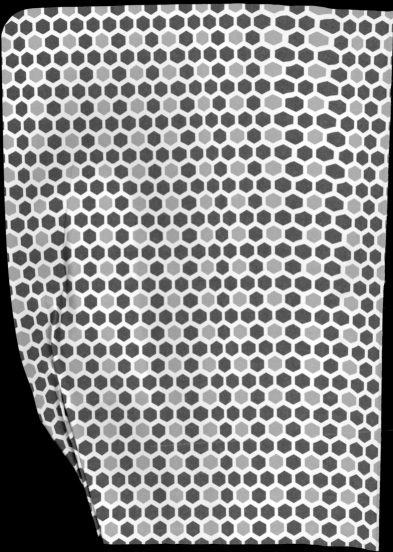